KU-497-777

INTELLECTUAL DISABILITY AND SOCIAL INCLUSION

A CRITICAL REVIEW

Edited by

Martin Bollard BSc(Hons) MA PGDip Ed RNLD
Senior Lecturer, Department of Social and Community Studies
Coventry University, Coventry, UK

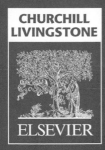

CHURCHILL
LIVINGSTONE

ELSEVIER

EDINBURGH LONDON NEW YORK OXFORD PHILADELPHIA ST LOUIS SYDNEY
TORONTO 2009

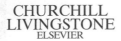

CHURCHILL
LIVINGSTONE
ELSEVIER

© 2009, Elsevier Limited. All rights reserved.

No part of this publication may be reproduced or transmitted in any form or by any means, electronic or mechanical, including photocopying, recording, or any information storage and retrieval system, without permission in writing from the publisher. Permissions may be sought directly from Elsevier's Rights Department: phone: (+1) 215 239 3804 (US) or (+44) 1865 843830 (UK); fax: (+44) 1865 853333; e-mail: healthpermissions@elsevier.com. You may also complete your request online via the Elsevierwebsite at http://www.elsevier.com/permissions.

First published 2009

ISBN 978 0 443 10418 3

British Library Cataloguing in Publication Data
A catalogue record for this book is available from the British Library

Library of Congress Cataloging in Publication Data
A catalog record for this book is available from the Library of Congress

Notice
Neither the Publisher nor the Editor assume any responsibility for any loss or injury and/or damage to persons or property arising out of or related to any use of the material contained in this book. It is the responsibility of the treating practitioner, relying on independent expertise and knowledge of the patient, to determine the best treatment and method of application for the patient.

The Publisher

ELSEVIER your source for books,
journals and multimedia
in the health sciences
www.elsevierhealth.com

Working together to grow
libraries in developing countries

www.elsevier.com | www.bookaid.org | www.sabre.org

 ELSEVIER   BOOK AID
International   Sabre Foundation

The
Publisher's
policy is to use
**paper manufactured
from sustainable forests**

Printed in China

Books are to be r

INTELLECTUAL DISABILITY
AND SOCIAL INCLUSION

362.
38

BOL

WITHDRAWN

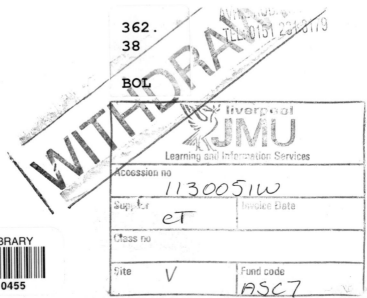

liverpool
JMU
Learning and Information Services

Accession no
1130051W

Supplier
eT

Invoice Date

Class no

Site
V

Fund code
ASC7

LIVERPOOL JMU LIBRARY

3 1111 01303 0455

For Elsevier:
Commissioning Editor: Steven Black, Mairi McCubbin
Development Editor: Sally Davies
Project Manager: Kerrie-Anne McKinlay
Designer: Erik Bigland
Illustration Manager: Gillian Richards
Illustrator: H.L. Studios

CONTENTS

Contents

FOREWORD

At the time of writing we are still waiting for the response of the Secretary of State for Health to the Michael Report. The report, which was published in the summer of 2008 highlighted the discrimination that people with intellectual disabilities suffer from mainstream health services. Whilst the report congratulated practitioners on some good examples of care, the general picture that was portrayed was extremely gloomy. The statistics painted an appalling picture of poor health and early death for many people with learning disabilities. The report gives examples of people with learning disabilities and carers not being listened to; people deemed unable to consent therefore being denied treatment; and diagnostic overshadowing in which symptoms that should be treated are seen as part of an individual's intellectual disability.

If this was the first inquiry of its kind then it would be bad enough. However it is merely the latest of a long line of reports that have drawn attention to discrimination against people with intellectual disabilities. People with long memories will remember the Ely Report that was published in 1969. The Ely inquiry investigated reports first printed in the News of the World and alleging abuse in a long stay hospital near Cardiff (HMSO, 1969). The report was the first in a long series of investigations that provided shocking material to a public that was largely ignorant of the conditions in long stay hospitals. The positive outcome was the gradual closure of the large long stay hospitals and the provision of community facilities to replace them. In many respects this heralded a new beginning for people with intellectual disabilities and the services set up for them. However, several reports indicate that there is still a long way to go. Recent examples such as the Cornwall investigation (Healthcare Commission, 2006), the Sutton and Merton investigation (Healthcare commission, 2007) , Mencap's Death by Indifference (Mencap, 2007) and the Disability Rights report (DRC, 2006) show that health services are still routinely depriving people with intellectual disabilities of good healthcare.

It seems that even when presented with the evidence that people's needs are not being met, the health service still finds it difficult to provide good care for people who have intellectual disabilities. Moreover it is likely that problems are not restricted to people with intellectual disabilities but to a range of those who do not fit the picture of a normal patient and therefore need extra time, more patience or a more imaginative means of communication. Health services need to change and adapt so that the best standards clearly evident in some places become the norm rather than the exception.

Whilst the health service needs to change, there are also changes with specialist learning disability services most of which are now organised through social care. Government policy for England has recently been formally refreshed and people with learning disabilities, their families and people working in services are trying to predict the impact of current and future trends. It seems that the settlement that was made at the time of hospital closure is now coming to end. That settlement included relatively well funded services supporting people living in shared housing. The evolving criteria assessments for fair access to care services, personalisation, individual budgets and the rhetoric of social inclusion have taken over in importance from concepts that those of us going through training in the eighties took for granted for so long: resettlement, normalisation and social role valorisation.

This book, for which I was delighted to be asked to write a forward, reflects this change and moves the debate on. As such it provides a thought provoking review. The editor has brought together a range of people who all have something significant to say about current services. Fittingly the book begins with a voice of someone with intellectual disabilities and then goes on to look at key aspects of current policy in different parts of the UK. The experience of people with learning disabilities in a changing world run throughout the book and this provides the overarching narrative.

I wish this book every success in promoting critical thinking about policy and practice in services for people with intellectual disabilities

Professor Duncan Mitchell
Manchester Metropolitan University and
Manchester Learning Disability Partnership.

DRC 2006 Equal Treatment: Closing the Gap. London, Disability Rights Commission.

Healthcare commission 2006 Joint Investigation Into Services for People with Learning Disabilities at Cornwall Partnership NHS Trust. London, Healthcare Commission.

Healthcare Commission 2007 Investigation into the Service for People with Learning Disability provided by the Sutton and Merton Primary Care Trust. London, Healthcare Commission.

HMSO 1969 Report of the Committee of Inquiry into Allegations of Ill Treatment of Patients and Other Irregularities at Ely Hospital Cardiff (Cmnd 3975). London, HMSO

Mencap 2007 Death by Indifference. Mencap, London.

PREFACE

This book focuses on the experience of people with intellectual disabilities across a number of different topics and issues that affect their lives. Within each chapter, the user experience and viewpoint has been presented in different ways – from focus groups, case studies, personal histories, narratives and general consultations. This collective user experience is married with the writers' expertise in their subject area. Other textbooks have started to recognise the importance of including the user voice in this way. This book aims to add to that body of knowledge and acknowledges that, for too long, accounts by people with intellectual disabilities themselves have been suppressed.

It is hoped that this book will be of use to all individuals involved with people with intellectual disabilities, particularly health and social care students, health and social care professionals, commissioners and policy makers.

People with intellectual disabilities are amongst one of the most socially excluded groups within society. They are a heterogeneous group of people with a diverse range of abilities and difficulties, with the majority of individuals living at home with their parents. Given such diversity and difference amongst this group of people, historically our understanding of disability has gone through many changes with varying opinions today as to what does and does not constitute an intellectual disability.

Taking a brief historical overview, the Poor Laws in 1601 sought to offer assistance to those in poverty, often as a result of a severe winter or a poor harvest, and provide the first indications of social policy and legislation being targeted at specific groups of people (McClimens 2005:29). The Poor Law Amendment Act (1834) established a way of classifying who was able-bodied and therefore able to contribute to the industrial focus of society at that time. The Poor Law Amendment Act (1834) also brought in a pluralistic provision of social, health and independent care for this group of people, with institutionalisation in the workhouses, relief by charitable organisations and self-help. This, coupled with the Victorian desire to 'medicalise' disability and deviance through its various Lunacy Acts (Pilgrim 1993), sought to isolate the individuals that were not economically productive by separating them on medical and pathological grounds (Oliver 1990). McClimens (2005:30) reminds us that this social construction of disability is a process of naming. Nowadays, for professionals working in the health and social care services this construct has centred on classifying people with a certain criterion and establishing whether individuals are eligible for a range of assistance and/or professional help.

More recent policy initiatives have sought to develop a more pluralistic and inclusive provision of care for people with intellectual disabilities. The desire to move away from 'long-stay' hospital provision, which originated in the Victorian era, was restated with the Better Services for the Mentally Handicapped Act (Department of Health and Social Services 1971) and has been given a broader and additional emphasis with the NHS Community Care Act (1990). The inclusive philosophy and desire to support the main-streaming of people with intellectual disabilities has been reiterated through *Valuing People* with less emphasis upon the necessity for specialist health ser-vices and 'inpatient' provision (Department of Health 2001). Indeed, the move away from a dependence on others, be that dependence on professionals or carers for all people with disabilities and other vulnerable groups, can be wit-nessed with the more recent political prominence given to self-directed forms of care, such as Direct Payments and Individual Budgets.

Individual Budgets are a key element in the present Government's ambi-tions for modernising social care (Glendinning et al 2006). An Individual Budget brings together the resources, both human and financial, from a num-ber of funding streams to in principle meet the personalised wishes of indi-viduals. This presents an opportunity for all people with disabilities and, importantly, people with intellectual disabilities (Armstrong 2002) to deter-mine their care needs. Although Individual Budgets have not been thoroughly evaluated yet, the process itself provides people with intellectual disabilities with a voice that has historically been denied.

This spirit of service-user involvement can be seen in the many other recent policy initiatives (Department of Health 2005, 2006). However, the extent to which people with intellectual disabilities themselves have been consulted regarding the impact of such policy initiatives is limited. This book attempts to remedy this and go beyond the impact that policy can have on people's lives, covering a range of topics that affect people with intellectual disabilities on a day-to-day basis.

Chapter 1 begins with an autobiographical account from Helena Frewin, a woman with intellectual disabilities. It includes some of her personal insights into different areas, many of which are the topics for the subsequent chapters in the book, thereby setting the scene for the book.

Chapter 2 takes a critical look at inclusion as a philosophy that has under-pinned many of the recent policy initiatives related to people with intellectual disabilities. I attempt to argue that the expectations that arise from dogmati-cally following inclusive endeavours need further empirical evaluation and would benefit from amalgamating other theories such as social capital. This is not to give prominence to either, but to highlight that it is worth considering how we build up the social capital of people with intellectual disabilities, in order that they may become potentially less segregated within society.

Chapters 3, 4 and 5 take a specific intellectual disability policy focus. The principle of inclusion is a key theme that runs through all of the policy directives across the United Kingdom. Chapter 3 examines *Valuing People* (Department of Health 2001), the first White Paper for thirty years on intellectual disability was bold and ambitious. John Turnbull reviews the legacy of the *Valuing People* document. He concludes that it is difficult to assess the true impact on the lives of people with intellectual disabilities as in many cases little evidence exists to assess the impact of *Valuing People* prior to its inception in 2001. However, greatest progress appears to be in person-centred planning and the least in developing more employment opportunities. Chapter 4 takes a Scottish policy perspective with a focus on *The Same as You* document. In this chapter, Michael Brown places the user perspective at the heart of his chapter. This chapter demonstrates how key members of the Scottish People First Movement have played an important part in influencing and developing this recent policy development for people with intellectual disabilities in Scotland. In Chapter 5, Owen Barr turns our attention to the policy initiative *Equal Lives*. This chapter particularly focuses upon the user involvement that led up to the production of the *Equal Lives* document and the subsequent user involvement that reviewed its impact. It reports on a key conference that sought the views of over a 100 users.

The difficulties that people with intellectual disabilities face when accessing mainstream health services are now well documented. Chapters 6, 7 and 8 explore these challenges with particular reference to mental health services, acute care and primary health care.

Chapter 6 by Dave Ferguson aims to describe the efforts, practice developments and service responses led by himself and his colleagues to promote an inclusive approach to service delivery and development. The narratives in this chapter are from people with intellectual disabilities and mental health issues.

Chapter 7 has been developed by Rick Robson and Ricky Owens, a man with intellectual disabilities who has extensive personal experience of the National Health Service. It offers insights into the difficulties faced when entering Acute Care. Solutions are put forward that may help to overcome the many difficulties that people with intellectual disabilities, their carers and health care workers face.

Chapter 8 by Susan Brady and Martin Bollard reports on two sets of findings from a primary health care project undertaken in Birmingham. The user and carer experiences of going to the doctor's are initially presented and then principally the user experience of health facilitation and Health Action Plans (HAP) in Birmingham is discussed.

Chapter 9 is written by Nick Fripp and Steve Day. It explores what leisure is from the perspective of a person with intellectual disabilities. The chapter is underpinned by a postmodernist standpoint, which provides a useful lens through which to consider leisure and this group of people. This is supported by substantial narratives from people with intellectual disabilities that are presented throughout the chapter.

Chapter 10 by Sarah Maguire is on the challenges faced by people with intellectual disabilities when trying to gain work. This chapter aims to examine barriers to employment, with a particular reference to employment and its effect on self-esteem, employers' perceptions of people with disabilities, the perceptions of individuals with intellectual disabilities about employment and the range of government initiatives to increase their employment opportunities. This chapter shares stories and views of people with intellectual disabilities about their own personal experience of the world of work.

In Chapter 11, Jackie Martin explores how further education courses can or cannot be accessed by people with intellectual disabilities. Elicited from a set of interviews with people with intellectual disabilities who attend further education courses, she highlights bullying and policy directives as barriers to inclusive further education.

Chapter 12 by Steven Rose gives a contemporary overview of the different types of housing options that are offered to people with intellectual disabilities. Through the use of case studies, the chapter shows the improvements made in the housing options available. The options discussed are the same as those on offer to many able-bodied individuals and have significantly shifted away from 'long-stay' hospital provision.

Ethnicity is a highly topical issue in modern Britain today and is the principal focus of Chapter 13 by Raghu Raghavan. Raghu ably shows through a number of user and carer case studies how people with intellectual disabilities from Black and Minority Ethnic (BME) communities can face distinct forms of marginalisation and disadvantage. This chapter concludes by calling for service agencies and practitioners to be more culturally sensitive and responsive to the needs of all BME communities and to actively engage with users and carers from such communities.

Chapter 14, by John Lahiff, explores some of the structural and philosophical challenges that underpin user involvement in higher education institutions. This chapter shows, through case studies, how a learning-disability nursing course within higher education has engaged people with intellectual disabilities in the development and delivery of the course itself.

Finally, Chapter 15, by Louise Talbott and Jane Parr, discusses the important issue of communication. The chapter writers propose an inclusive communication approach and share some practical examples of an inclusive communication model from their experience as therapists who are employed within a Specialist NHS Speech and Language Therapy Service.

REFERENCES

Armstrong D 2002 The politics of self-advocacy and people with learning disabilities. Policy and Politics 20:196-213.

Department of Health 1990 The NHS and Community Act. HMSO, London.

Department of Health 2001 Valuing People: a strategy for people with learning disabilities for the 21st century. HMSO, London.

Department of Health 2005 Independence, wellbeing and choice our vision for the future of adult social care. Department of Health, London.

Department of Health 2006 Our health, our care, our say. CM 6737. The Stationery Office, London.

Department of Health and Social Services 1971 Better services for the mentally handicapped. HMSO, London.

Glendinning C, Challis D, Fernandez J L et al 2006 Evaluating the individual budget pilot projects. Research note. Journal of Care Services Management 1(2):123-128.

McClimens A 2005 From vagabonds to Victorian values, the social construction of disability identity. In: Grant G et al (eds) Learning disability: a life cycle approach to valuing people. Open University Press.

Oliver M 1990 The politics of disablement. Macmillan, London.

Pilgrim D 1993 Anthology: policy. In: Bornat J et al (eds) Community care: a reader. Macmillan, London.

Martin Bollard
Coventry, 2009

CONTRIBUTORS

Owen Barr BSc(Hons) MSc PhD RGN RNLD CNLD RNT
Head of School, School of Nursing, University of Ulster, Derry,
Northern Ireland; Editor, *Journal of Intellectual Disabilities*

Martin Bollard BSc(Hons) MA PG Dip Ed RNLD
Senior Lecturer, Department of Social and Community Studies,
Coventry University, Coventry, UK

Susan Brady RNMH PGCert PGDip MSc Advanced Practice in Nursing
Clinical Lead for Health Facilitation, South Birmingham Primary Care
NHS Trust, Birmingham, UK

Michael Brown BSc(Hons) MSc PGCE Dip CMHC Dip Prof Stds Cert CPT
RGN RNLD
Lecturer, School of Nursing, Midwifery and Social Care,
Napier University, Edinburgh, UK; Nurse Consultant, NHS Lothian,
Edinburgh, UK

Steve Day MSc CSS
Assistant Director, Brandon Trust, Bristol, UK

Dave Ferguson BNS(Hons) MA RNLD CNLD CPT
Nurse Consultant, Mental Health in Learning Disability and
Academic Practitioner, Hampshire Partnership NHS Trust and
University of Southampton, Southampton, UK

Helena Frewin
Director, Thera Trust, Nottingham, UK

Nick Fripp MSc (Leadership of Public Services) MSc (Interprofessional
Studies LD) DipRSA
Head of Operational Transformation, Cornwall County Council and
Cornwall Partnership NHS Trust, Truro, UK

John Lahiff BSc(Hons) CertEd RN
Senior Lecturer, Department of Social and Community Studies,
Coventry University, Coventry, UK

Sarah Maguire BA(Hons) MA CIPD
Director, Organisational Support, Choice Support, London, UK

Jackie Martin BA(Hons) MA PGCE DipSW
Senior Lecturer, Division of Social Work and Health Studies,
De Montfort University, Leicester, UK

Ricky Owens
Health Advisor, Department of Health Valuing People Support Team, UK

Jane Parr CertMRCSLT
Clinical Lead, Speech and Language Therapy, Leicester Frith Hospital,
Leicester; Lead, Communication Strategy, Leicester, Leicestershire and
Rutland, UK

Raghu Raghavan BA MSc PGCE RNLD PhD
Reader, School of Nursing, School of Health, Education and
Community Studies, Northumbria University, Newcastle-upon-Tyne, UK

Rick Robson RN DipN(Lond) ENB N45
Senior Nurse (Learning Disabilities), South Staffordshire and Shropshire
Health Care NHS Foundation Trust; Chair, National A2A Network; Chair,
West Midlands National Learning Disability Nursing Network, UK

Steven Rose MSc RNLD RMN FRSA
Chief Executive, Choice Support, London, UK

Louise Talbott BSc
Senior Specialist Speech and Language Therapist, Leicestershire Partnership
NHS Trust, Oakham, UK

John Turnbull BA MSc PhD RNLD
Director of Nursing and Quality Performance, Ridgeway Partnership,
Oxfordshire Learning Disability, NHS Trust; Visiting Professor,
University of Northampton, Northampton, UK

Contributors

One story

Helena Frewin

Helena is an able woman with intellectual disabilities who I have had the pleasure of working with on a number of occasions, prior to the development of this chapter. This chapter represents a long-term aspiration of Helena's to share her own experiences, in her own way. It is the culmination of work that has taken place between Helena and myself over the last 18 months, sitting in her front room listening and typing up what she has to say. It is therefore seen as a discursive life story (Plummer 2001). In line with Helena's wishes, I have in no way interpreted what Helena has said. I have not attempted to analyse what she has narrated or reflected on in any specific way. I have only suggested areas that Helena may wish to talk about that are in line with the rest of the chapters presented within the book and may be covered in other life story interviews.

It's normal to be different. No-one is the same. We all have our own little quirks. We have our different opinions which are often made of people within five minutes of meeting them.

Everyone has different ways of communicating. This does not just include speech. People's facial expressions are a form of communication. People can see if you are happy or sad, or feeling angry. Sometimes people cannot speak so they rely on these forms of communication. We rely on all four of the senses, hearing, touch sight and smell. If you lose one or more of these, as I have, the other senses have to compensate.

MY FAMILY

My mum did not know she was pregnant and she did not know she was carrying a virus. I was born in a little county hospital near to where my mum and dad lived. I was born with a hole in my heart. I lost total sight in one eye and I am partially sighted in the other. When I was very little because the county hospital did not have the equipment to help me, they moved me to a city hospital in London where more could be done.

I had a hundred heart attacks and a lot of operations and I was in and out of hospital until I was eight, with a lot of hospital appointments until I was about twelve. I did not start nursery school until I was eight. I do not remember too much about it, apart from having milk at break times, singing songs and saying the Lord's Prayer. When I was a little older I changed classes and started doing Maths and English. At eleven I went in a taxi to school with three other children. I am still friends with Beth now. She used to live close to me. I used to sing songs in the taxi with Beth but Beth went to a different school. Beth did not like her school and neither did I, as I was bullied by a younger but taller girl than me.

I have a sister and there always seemed to be a competition between us. I often felt that I missed out on conversations and did not feel I fitted in. My mum and dad were teachers and, when I was unwell, they had to stay off work and spend time at the hospital with me. When my sister went to university, it made me feel different as I think that I would never have the opportunity to go to university.

After school I went away to college. This was a difficult time and I felt that there was a conspiracy between the head teacher and the social worker. My parents got in touch with a social worker. I wanted to live in the area near to my parents. I moved in with my parents for a while and then the social worker showed me around some new places to live. Some were not suitable but the social worker went through all the options. A little while later I got a phone call from the social worker to look at some new sheltered housing. Unknown to the social worker I had put my name down on the housing waiting list. A week before I was due to move into the sheltered houses that the social worker had found for me, I got a telephone call from the council saying a house had come up for me. Unfortunately I was not in a position to take up this option.

SCHOOL TIMES

Children start to learn from an early age. When you get to the dreaded school age, which is just as bad for the parents as it is for the children, it can be difficult. I remember the times my mum waved me off at the gate and my dad drops me off at the school disco and insists that he will pick you up afterwards – it is so embarrassing! Then you have exams to go through, all the stress.

EMPLOYMENT

My first work opportunity was when I worked on the Fair Deal management committee. I helped out in meetings that looked at the future of Fair Deal as an advocacy organisation and also edited their newsletter.

My existing job was advertised in a number of papers and my friend told me through my person centred plan. It was to support the organisation, Thera Trust in the East Midlands, as a part time Service Director, to mainly chair meetings. I also take part in board meetings but I find that difficult so I am having a personal assistant, but Thera want me to have one that I could choose.

My first interview for this job was at Derby with a presentation and number of people talking at me. There were 40 people who went through to the workshop stage after the first interview. We had various exercises that we had to do to tell us what a service director did and this took all day. Two days later I found out but the bit between the first and second interview was long. I applied for the job in my own right not because of my disability and I am really pleased that I got the job.

Because of my experience of this interview, I could talk about the Managing Director's (for a person with intellectual disabilities) post and how to organise the interviews. The whole purpose of my job is to talk to members with intellectual disabilities who use Thera Trust. One of my objectives within Thera was to look at the benefit issues that can stop people with intellectual disabilities getting jobs. Two weeks after my new job started my benefits stopped. Luckily I had money in savings but many people will not have that opportunity.

FURTHER EDUCATION

I have done two courses at further education colleges. The first one I did on independent living (money skills, cooking and basic English) with other people with intellectual disabilities.

The second course that I did was on computing skills, computer software and that has been beneficial for my current job. I would also say to colleges they should make their courses accessible and relevant courses on getting a job, independent living, leisure and social skills. Leisure and social skills involve knowing how to make friends with people, solve arguments, how to behave appropriately. Unfortunately, it is too late after school but these skills are particularly important. I heard the Prime Minister talk about responsibility and people with intellectual disabilities need to take responsibility for their actions and lives, although this is difficult for some and easy for others. If people find it hard to take responsibility then it is up to the support services to help them.

I think it is important that people with intellectual disabilities are engaged with politics but the politicians should engage with our lives. If they want our vote they should listen to us. I am more convinced by the current Prime Minister than I was by Tony and I was quite convinced by Tony.

LEISURE

Leisure is non-existent for me. Well, I do go swimming but that is about it. I go into town and go out for coffee with friends. I always think I should invite more friends around.

Friends and relationships – I don't have many friends but the friends I have are close. They live nearby which helps. The thing about this is that lots of people with intellectual disabilities have few friends just like people without disabilities.

I am trying to look more generally at using the gym myself and working with the local gym to see if they can provide the support to people with intellectual disabilities.

In terms of money, I personally have had a direct payment as there was not anyone locally to give the right kind of support. A direct payment would give you the choice to choose the person to work with you at the time you want the support. The big thing is about choice. Individual Budgets, I don't know, IB is another word for direct payments, I think Individual Budgets are controlled by social services and it is very difficult to have the whole control yourself as with direct payments. I still get Disability Living Allowance, Care and Mobility component, which helps.

HEALTH

Generally I am fit and healthy, I have not been to the doctors or the hospital for ages. Coming back to politics I think inclusion is more than going to the doctors, it is about them having greater understanding of intellectual disabilities. For someone with autism it is stressful waiting in the waiting room or for an appointment at the hospital. Training is needed for doctors who are practising now as well as medical students. I have done lots of doctor training through the university and through Mencap.

Talking to them about my life has a lot of benefit to the medical students. I talked to them about my heart and eyesight difficulties that I have had in the past, but the work with Mencap it was with carers as well, in order to give the carer perspective to students. A group of third year students remembered me from when they were first year students. It made me feel good and how beneficial explaining our lives can be for all students.

HOUSING

I live by myself in a rented one bed-roomed flat. I have lived on my own for 3.5 years. It is good to live by yourself to have your own choices, to choose what food you want to eat. There are disadvantages, cooking, cleaning and it gets quite lonely only me. One day I would like to have a shared ownership scheme, where you own a percentage of the house and you rent it from the housing association. I am starting to look into this more through my current work. I do not know enough about the different housing, but in an attempt to change from a sheltered housing scheme, where three houses were knocked into one into a supported living scheme, I felt it difficult to work by just having the same staff. I did not at the time think that this would make any difference. Sheltered housing is where you are more independent and responsible for paying your own bills. Residential, I suppose a lot more gets done for you. There are more regulations for residential homes.

POLICY

Valuing People did not do what it needed to do, it was all really exciting but has not lived up to the expectations. I do not know how effective it has been having people with intellectual disabilities on Partnerships Boards. From my own experience, I should say for me sometimes I felt that I was not making a difference because the changes that I suggested were not always acted upon. Towards the end, a huge effort was made focusing on how the Board communicated with all people with intellectual disabilities and outside with other people with intellectual disabilities. I did feel like I was an equal member of the Board and it is really important that people with intellectual disabilities have a voice.

My aspirations for the future are for the Government to take more responsibility for helping us access services, particularly health and further education.

As part of that the more people with intellectual disabilities need to have the opportunity to tell their stories to help others understand what our lives are about.

REFERENCE

Plummer K 2001 The call of life stories in ethnographic research. In: Atkinson P, Coffey A, Delmont S et al (eds) Handbook of ethnography. Sage, London.

A review and critique

Martin Bollard

Social inclusion has been given significant emphasis within public policy and as an underpinning philosophy to guide the improvement of the lives of people with intellectual disabilities. The goal for social inclusion activists is, in some cases, to ensure people with intellectual disabilities have full and equal access to health care, social roles and relationships that are equal to their non-disabled partners.

This chapter aims to argue that social inclusion, adopted as a single concept to improve the lives of people with intellectual disabilities, is in danger of being mere ideological rhetoric unless seen in conjunction with the broader concept of social capital. Putnam (2000) conceptualises social capital theory as aspects of social organisation such as interpersonal trust, norms of reciprocity, social engagement that can foster community and social participation. Secondly, the chapter aims to highlight that to make real changes for people with intellectual disabilities, it is necessary to merge inclusive theory with a social capital perspective. The perception of people with intellectual disabilities by others is as important a factor as their individual capacity to contribute to communities (Bates & Davies 2004). Assisting those individuals with intellectual disabilities who wish to forge relationships and networks outside of the intellectual disability community may, through the acceptance of others, provide a platform for a more inclusive life.

The chapter claims that it is unfair and raises unrealistic expectations to pursue policy directives that are dogmatically underpinned by social inclusion theories without the consideration of other theories, such as social capital and further empirical evaluation. Social capital, it is claimed, has captured the imagination of social scientists worldwide (Halpern 2005). Both social inclusion and social capital, as theoretical concepts, require further empirical evaluation not only as terms in their own right, but more importantly when associated with people with intellectual disabilities.

Case studies are presented to help merge the two concepts of social inclusion and social capital. The case studies are drawn from a primary care project that I lead in the West Midlands during the late 1990s and have not been published elsewhere.

To contextualise the chapter, it is deemed initially necessary to provide an overview of disability.

To date a number of authoritative arguments have been put forward that can help develop our understanding of disability (Bury 1997, Oliver 1996, Shakespeare 2006).

Without doubt, Mike Oliver's work has helped ground and promote the disability movement. This work has sought to move thinking away from the personal/physical difficulties associated with the impairment/disability discourse and focus the attention upon the social barriers that exist for many people with disabilities. Shakespeare (2006) refutes this, claiming it is unrealistic to neglect the real impact that the impairment has on the lives of many people with disabilities. One of the useful arguments put forward by Shakespeare (2006), that can crystallize our comprehension of disability, is the necessity, as he sees it, to cut through the binary distinctions of impairment and disability. In other words it is too simple to distinguish disability as either a physical or social problem and what is important is to establish what people with disabilities themselves consider most impacts upon their lives. What can further complicate a genuine understanding of disability is the dichotomy of the social model versus the medical model. Within the UK for too long Shakespeare (2006:10) argues the social model has been seen as the right way and the medical model as the wrong way.

Bury (1999) and Williams (1999) consider disability differently to these latter perspectives. Bury (1997) argues that the International Classification of Impairment Disabilities and Handicaps (ICIDH) has defined this set of terms individually and distinctly (Impairment, Disability and Handicap), which in turn has influenced the World Health Organization (1980) definitions. Importantly, Bury (1997) claims those terms are far from being associated with an oppressive medical model; in fact the ICIDH classifications have benefited the lives of people with disabilities. Such an argument is based upon a resistance to the 'over socialized social model' and as Bury (1997) states perceiving disability as a relational concept. Williams (1999) parts company with the original disability theorists, such as Mike Oliver, believing they attempt to ignore the reality of impairment through a social model of oppression. A realistic perspective perceives disability as an 'emergent property', one that acknowledges the interplay between the biological reality of impairment – structural conditioning (enablement and constraints) and socio-cultural interaction (Williams 1999).

The crux of the argument advocated by Shakespeare (2006) is that for the last 40 years, social scientists and campaigners everywhere have regarded disability as being bound up in the social context, with a particular emphasis on the disadvantage, the social exclusion and the oppression experienced by many disabled people. Given this, there has been too much conceptualising of disability and not enough emphasis placed upon research from the perspective of people with disabilities themselves (Shakespeare 2006).

Scholars such as Michael Bury (2000) have attempted to make room for the experiences of people with disabilities:

'Our aim it will be remembered was to challenge the medical model and the assumptions about disablement. Most importantly, our aim was to bring handicap onto the health care agenda. That is, we were pressing for greater recognition of (what came to be called) the social exclusion in response to disablement.'

Bury 2000:1074

Thomas (2004) argues that over time a social relational model of disability has been lost (one based on Finkelstein & Hunt's original work in the 1970s), with the prominence of the social model. Thomas (1999) advocates a rediscovering of a social relational understanding of disability. Disability is a form of social oppression involving the social imposition of restrictions of activity on people with impairments and the socially engendered undermining of their psycho-emotional well being (Thomas 1999:60). Although Thomas (1999) talks about revisiting the concept of a social relational perspective of disability, based upon her work with disabled women, a broad approach to understand the interplay of social relationships and caring environments that constitute the lived experience of all people with disabilities is required. Shakespeare (2006) argues that disability is always an interaction between the individual and structural factors; this necessitates a holistic understanding that does not get too focused upon defining disability as a deficit or a structural disadvantage.

PEOPLE WITH INTELLECTUAL DISABILITIES

The acknowledgement that individuals' difficulties arise from their impairment has been reflected in the core business of specialist health services established to support and rehabilitate people with intellectual disabilities for the last three decades (Royal College of Nursing 1980, Department of Health 1998, 2000, 2001, 2007a). These services have been built upon the claim that people with intellectual disabilities are entitled to special assistance (Redley & Weinburg 2007). Drawn from a lucid ethnographic study, Redley & Weinburg (2007) highlight the key tension between, on the one hand the political aspiration of pursing an inclusion project (*Valuing People*) that is based on the promotion of rights, choice and independence and articulated through issues related to participation and the often perceived contrary position that is demonstrated in the professional recognition of need. The latter perspective should not eclipse the other.

Health is a broad and dynamic concept and one that if viewed holistically can impact on many aspects of the lives of all individuals. Similar to other vulnerable groups of people, people with intellectual disabilities often have unrecognised and unmet health needs (Beange 2000) and the social determinants that impact on their individual health can be complex. As with everyone, the ability to enjoy leisure, recreational and social pursuits can be restricted, if individual health difficulties are present. Conversely, the impact that social factors and psychosocial stress can have on individual health and well being has been acknowledged (Wilkinson 1996). Working towards a true understanding of the needs of people with intellectual disabilities therefore requires a sensitive and professional mediation through what have traditionally been seen as health and social care needs. Perceiving need in this dualistic way does not reflect the complexity of needs that many people with intellectual disabilities have.

A review and critique

The recent reports *Equal treatment: closing the gap* (Disability Rights Commission 2006) and *Death by indifference* (Mencap 2007) demonstrate that people with intellectual disabilities can highlight the limitations within the National Health Service. Whether the evidence drawn from these reports represents wider societal discrimination against people with intellectual disabilities is not yet fully substantiated by people with intellectual disabilities themselves or researchers. The reports do highlight that people with intellectual disabilities can be excluded and discriminated against when seeking mainstream health care and in many cases their basic rights to mainstream health care are not always upheld.

Many people with disabilities strive for a life that involves meaningful paid employment, yet less than 10% of people with intellectual disabilities are in employment and the employment rates for this group of people have not changed for the last 7 years (Department of Health 2007c). This presents a conflict for people with intellectual disabilities within a knowledge base society (Brown & Lauder 2000) that on the one hand demands individual agents to seek out training and employment opportunities for themselves, compared with their intellectual difficulties that can require support and assistance to achieve college places and employment opportunities.

SOCIAL INCLUSION

People with intellectual disabilities are among one of the most socially disadvantaged groups of people within society (Disability Rights Commission 2006). Many people with intellectual disabilities have a complexity of health and well being difficulties that at times makes it a challenge for them to be included in the day to day activities of life, which many non-disabled people enjoy.

Although evidence of how people with intellectual disabilities have been excluded predates the present Labour Government, the conception of the Social Exclusion Unit within that administration heavily politicised the desire to remove social barriers that put many vulnerable groups on the margins of society (Byrne 2005). The term exclusion was quickly replaced by inclusion within political circles. The 'New Labour' objective for greater social inclusion and cohesion is founded on the claim that capitalist societies, by their very nature, create inequalities and conflicts of interests (Byrne 2005). Fairclough (2000) argues that the objective of social inclusion proposes a contrasting standpoint:

> 'By focusing on those who are excluded from society and the ways of including them, shifts away the inequalities and conflicts of interest amongst those who are included and presupposes that there is nothing inherently wrong with contemporary society as long as it is made more inclusive through government policies.'
>
> Fairclough 2000:65

Inclusion, in this context, becomes an ideology, ideology being referred to as an idea or set of ideas that forms the basis for a political way of thinking (Oxford Dictionary 1997).

Labonte (2004) argues that the twinned concepts of social inclusion and social exclusion are the latest constructs to be heralded by practitioners, researchers and policy makers. Adopting such conceptual terms, like their predecessors social capital and social cohesion, without critical examination of the premises that underpin them, presents risks (Labonte 2004).

Many individuals with intellectual disabilities are routinely subordinated to perform ancillary roles in day to day decision making processes (Armstrong 2002). Moreover, the reality for many people with intellectual disabilities is that they find themselves excluded and often powerless and therefore have to campaign for their 'rights' under the umbrella of self advocacy movements such as *People First*.

Without recognising the structures and systems that have excluded people in the first place, it is difficult to carefully plan and consider how individuals may have sustained inclusion in their communities. Although important aspects that impact upon the lives of people with intellectual disabilities, this debate goes beyond the material inequalities that many people with disabilities experience. This discussion is centred on whether there are the sufficient conditions within communities for people with intellectual disabilities to fully participate. In addition to this, can people with intellectual disabilities be supported ably enough for their presence within such communities to be recognised and valued?

Many people with intellectual disabilities often aspire to be more socially included (McConkey 2007). Studies have documented the reduced access to community facilities and the lack of friendships that people with intellectual disabilities have (Myers et al 1998). The isolation associated with former institutionalised practices has been widely documented (Emerson & Hatton 1996). Similarly, the impact of limited engagement with others that is associated with campus/congregated living is well known (Department of Health 2001).

As more and more individuals are re-patronised to live, in many cases closer to their relatives, the opportunities for the development of more self-directed forms of care such as direct payments and individual budgets increase. Such forms of care that transfer the monies from local authorities and the decision making for welfare back to the individual and their carers present opportunities for personalised care (Department of Health 2007c). This process can provide people with disabilities, and other vulnerable groups, the opportunity to choose and potentially engage with their communities.

SOCIAL CAPITAL

Social capital predates social inclusion as a concept that attempts to understand how social networks and communities organise and pull themselves together based on a set on mutual goals. The concept itself has been largely attributed to three different writers. Initially Pierre Bourdieu, whose early work in the 1960s and 1970s sought to establish culture as a dynamic and creative, but also structured, phenomenon. Baron et al (2000) claim that the notion of social capital evolved for Bourdieu from his interest in an array of other forms of capital, such as economic, cultural, linguistic and scholastic.

James Coleman, another seminal social capital theorist, focused his work on the relationship between educational achievement and social inequality (Coleman 1988). Later Coleman further elaborated on his work:

'Social capital is a set of resources that inhere in family relations and in community social organisation and that are useful for the cognitive or social development of a child and young person.'

Coleman 1994:300

The third and more recent writer on social capital is Robert Putnam. Putnam (1995:2000) conceptualises social capital theory as aspects of social organisation such as interpersonal trust, norms of reciprocity, social engagement that can foster community and social participation. Carpiano (2007) argues that studies of social capital have almost exclusively relied upon Putnam's thesis. Bates & Davies (2004) suggest that the concept itself has a utility for human services. It is also suggested that the relationship between social capital and social inclusion is reciprocal. The inclusion advocates who are working with people with intellectual disabilities can promote the social capital in whole communities, not solely for the service users themselves (Bates & Davies 2004).

David Halpern (2005) argues that social capital has caught the imagination of scholars and policy makers worldwide. For some scholars it is the most significant concept within the social sciences for 50 years and David Halpern describes social capital as:

'Social networks and the norms that govern their character – it is valued for its potential to facilitate individual and community action, especially through the solution of collective problems.'

Halpern 2005:4

Drawn from the extensive work by Putnam (2000), two types of social capital emerge. Bridging social capital, which is outward-looking and inclusive, and bonding social capital, which is inward-looking and exclusive. Bridging social capital attempts to connect people across social divides. The Disability Movement in the 1970s and the politically active work undertaken by organisations such as UPIAS are examples of how disabled people have expressed their 'rights' and aspirations and have fought hard to gain collective recognition for their needs. Bonding social capital reiterates exclusive identities and homogenous groups. This can be demonstrated by ethnic groups and collectives such as the National Childbirth Trust support groups. Therefore being an active part of an organisation allows people to feel more connected with the larger society. Bridging social capital is important to the success of a civil society, with integral benefits for individuals, communities and societies (Islam et al 2006).

Whether social capital can promote the health of communities is not yet established. The study by Capriano (2007) tests a set of neighbourhood conditions and social capital with adult health behaviours. The conditions are predominantly linked to the work of Pierre Bourdieu, stressing the human and social resources necessary within social networks to make the networks useful. In this context, social capital refers to the following four areas:

- Social support (the people support systems that individuals can draw upon to help them cope with their daily lives)
- Social leverage (the support necessary to help individuals access information, survive financially and even to advance themselves)

- Informal social control concerns (the ability of the local community/neighbourhood to keep itself safe and free from criminal activity)
- Neighbourhood organisation participation (a collective neighbourhood action group to respond to neighbourhood issues).

This study showed that specific forms of social capital can be both negatively and positively associated with promoting health outcomes and that further research in this area should account for the different types of social capital resources that arise within community networks, not simply focusing on the mutual values that bind such networks together (Capriano 2007).

Given the extensive variables involved, measuring 'real' improvements in a population's health and well being is complex. Portes (1998) has attempted to clarify the origins of social capital and points to differences between individual social capital and social capital associated with a social community. Folland (2007) claims that on the whole when social capital is robustly tested against a set of indicators, that is based on the work of Robert Putnam (2000), then cases of social capital can improve health. Nonetheless, social capital, as a conceptual framework, is clearly not a panacea to developing a greater understanding of what can or cannot improve the health of communities. Riddell et al (1997) provide a positive perspective of where, if social capital is seen to include all members of society, further inclusion of people with intellectual disabilities into the workplace, for example, could increase the circulation and accumulation of social capital within communities. It is at this point that the goals of social capitalist and inclusion advocates are intertwined.

Other forms of capital

The concept of social capital has emerged within the intellectual disability field with some popularity at the same time as Valuing People (Department of Health 2001) required social inclusion to underpin the development of intellectual disability services (Bates & Davies 2004). Other forms of capital, in particular human capital, are worth referring to in relation to people with intellectual disabilities. Many people with intellectual disabilities are taking on different forms of employment and volunteering. These employment options may not be financially rewarded by the national average salary of £26 000, nonetheless they offer this group of people opportunities to develop their human capital. There are no clear definitions as to what personable attributes should be included in a definition of human capital (Halpern 2005). Halpern (2005:15) offers a definition of human capital as being:

> 'Stocks of expertise accumulated by a worker – knowing how to do
> something, for example, a professional training. It is valued for
> its income earning potential in the future.'

Moreover, it is helpful to define social capital as something formed from human relationships (Folland 2006). People with intellectual disabilities themselves have stated that the reduced opportunity to form meaningful relationships can affect their mental health for instance (Hardy et al 2006).

A review and critique

For the purposes of this chapter and given that this group of people often have limited social networks, isolated from family members, human capital will be highlighted as an important feature to consider in a debate that is concerned with the inclusion of a marginalised group of people. Human capital can be seen as the decision to build up an individual's skills and knowledge as a personal investment in their future (Pavey 2006). Hancock sees the concept more broadly encompassing features of:

> 'Healthy, well educated, well skilled, innovative and creative people who are engaged in their communities and participate in governance.'
>
> Hancock 2001:276

The very nature of having an intellectual disability may for some people reduce the potential to develop such aspects of human capital. Furthermore if we apply a universal understanding of human capital, as being an individual's skills, qualifications and length of schooling (Baron et al 2000), then this group of people could be easily excluded altogether within a learning society that configures itself around the necessity for skills acquisition and qualifications (Brown & Lauder 2000). However, there are other skills and human potential that people with intellectual disabilities have that can be valued for example in the employment arena (see Chapter 10 by Sarah Maguire). Through gaining employment, there are examples of where people with intellectual disabilities have developed their entrepreneurial skills (Marshall 2006) and the acclaimed film Bread Makers, which shows how 12 people with intellectual disabilities work in Garvald Bakery, Edinburgh (www.guardian.co.uk/society/2008/jan16/learning disability), highlights this further.

APPLYING SOCIAL INCLUSION AND SOCIAL CAPITAL THEORIES

Case study 2.1

George is a 43-year-old man with a mild intellectual disability. He lives in a self-contained flat in a socially deprived part of the city. He has no living relatives and has no close friendships. He regularly attends the local 'drop-in centre' for people with intellectual disabilities. This provides him with people to meet with but with whom on most occasions he does not really like.

George is not interested in keeping his flat tidy or clean. There are many pots and pans that have been left in his sink for days. He can cook himself small meals, but finds it easier to rely on take away meals and frozen food that he can cook in the microwave. Generally George himself is clean and tidy although he finds using his washing machine difficult, due to an arthritic right hand, his dominant hand.

George is morbidly obese and although he walks and catches the bus on a regular basis, he has recently been complaining of a shortness of breath. His feet and ankles are swollen and he frequently attends his GP practice, where he is well known. George himself is beginning to recognise that he is attending unnecessarily. His GP is generally sensitive and supportive and has been trying to suggest that he loses some weight. His doctor prescribed a 'prescription for sport' last year, which entitled him to free membership at the local gym. George felt uncomfortable using the gym and only went once. He felt unsafe using the gym at night and while walking back to the bus stop by himself through the city centre.

George likes the Practice Nurse and every time he goes to the doctors he invariably ends up seeing the nurse. Dawn, the Practice Nurse, has recently got George started on a course of hypertensive medication, but is concerned about his 'inactivity' during the day as she feels it is affecting his health. George tells her that he feels fine and does not need any help as he walks everywhere.

More recently with the document *Progress to transformation* (Department of Health 2007b) the ambition of inclusion is reiterated for people with learning disabilities with a set of priorities:

- Personalisation – to enable people to have real choice and control over their lives and services
- What people do during the day (evenings and weekends) – helping people to be properly included in their communities, with a particular focus on paid work
- Better health – ensuring that the National Health Service provides full and equal access to good quality health care
- Access to housing that people want and need – with a particular emphasis on home ownership and tenancies
- Making sure that change happens and the policy is delivered – including making Partnership Boards more effective (Department of Health 2007:11).

Indicators of social inclusion have been highlighted elsewhere (Emerson & McVilly 2004):

1. The number of friends outside of the home; defined as people whom the individual meets on a regular basis and shared activities; who confide in and provide support for one another.
2. The number of neighbours in the area who know the individual by name or who are known by the individual.
3. The frequency of contact with their family during the past month.

Against these three indicators, George could be judged to have a poor level of social inclusion, with no friends or relatives and only some regular contact through a 'drop-in centre'. When George has sought opportunities to increase his social network by attending a gym, he has felt uncomfortable and unsafe. People with intellectual disabilities living in fear and feeling unsure of who to trust has been reported elsewhere (Mencap 1999).

The only regular contact George has is with the Practice Nurse, a health professional who is primarily concerned with his obesity and weight reduction. The intellectual disability nurse is well placed to offer health advice and support the practice nurse (Department of Health 2007:25), however the Practice Nurse at the time was unaware that an intellectual disability nurse existed to help with people like George. Any professional review of George is likely to prioritize his health needs, given his morbid obesity, before considering his apparent exclusion for social activities, thereby placing the emphasis on the impairment over the disability. George himself has stated that he does not really like the people at the drop-in centre, therefore attempts to build up his social capital and 'inclusivity' would go against his wishes. The necessity to be person-centred and responsive to service users has been given unprecedented publicity through policy directives (Department of Health 2000, 2006) and professional regulating bodies (NMC, CCETSW). Moreover, in this case there was limited professional knowledge regarding the appropriate services that may have been available to access and present a choice to George. Attempts to meet the needs of George more substantially would require the merger of inclusive strategies and social capital endeavours' to bridge and bond relationships for people like George (Putnam 2000).

Case study 2.2

Jenny is a 28-year-old woman with a moderate intellectual disability who lives with her mum and sister. Jenny has a good sense of humour and is loved dearly by her sister Janet. Her sister has a mild intellectual disability and is 3 years older than her. They have no other friends or relatives who live nearby. Jenny and Janet used to attend the local day centre for people with intellectual disabilities until it closed a few years ago. They spend most of their time helping their mum with the shopping and running their house. They both enjoy their food but their mum has recently become concerned about the amount of weight they have both put on. Jenny and Janet were invited to their local doctor's surgery to have a health check. The health check comprised a 34-itemised review, covering health, social and well being questions. Jenny and Janet are both short in stature but have no reported health difficulties. The health check revealed a Body Mass Index of 43 and 45 respectively for Jenny and Joan (Jenny was 18 stone and Joan was 18 and a half stone in weight). The Practice Nurse who undertook the health check recommended that they both try and lose some weight. Their mum was unsure about how to go about this. On the back of the health check was the name of a local dietician who worked with adults with intellectual disabilities. After some initial reluctance from their GP to refer Jenny and Janet to the dietician (the GP was unsure as to whether Jenny and Janet would be able to follow a weight management programme), he agreed to refer them both. Jenny and Janet worked well with the dietician. The programme helped their mum review their diet, monitor and record their weight on a regular basis and generally raised awareness of the different food types for the family. The dietician also encouraged Jenny and Janet to take up a form of exercise that they enjoyed. Their mum recommended swimming as it was an activity the girls had enjoyed when they were young.

Jenny and Janet joined the local sports centre that has a lovely swimming pool and went there three times a week. They became friendly with the staff and started joining in other exercise classes that were run there. This has been the biggest gain for both Jenny and Janet. They feel happy going there and feel they belong there. After 6 months, the dietician weighed Jenny and Janet. They had each lost over 3 stone and are able to consider what they both now eat. The mum told the dietician that they are like two different people.

Using the same social inclusion indicators (Emerson & McViffey 2004), Jenny and Janet have a higher level of social inclusion than George. They are members of a close knit family but still have limited scope to develop relationships outside of their family circle. The health check was a catalyst to improve the health and well being of both Jenny and Janet. The necessity for primary care to adopt a regular health assessment for people with intellectual disabilities has been well documented (Disability Rights Commission 2006, Department of Health 2007). The support of the specialist dietitian was instrumental in not only achieving weight loss but encouraging the two sisters to make lifestyle changes. The relationships formed with staff at the sports centre has improved both individual and community social capital for Jenny and Janet (Portes 1998). Their sense of belonging to the sports centre has allowed them to bridge the gap between the non-disabled and themselves as women with intellectual disabilities. Furthermore, the sports centre as a social organisation has embraced the two sisters and they now share a bond (Putnam 2000) to improve individual health and well being. In this case, the social inclusion achieved by Jenny and Janet has more meaning through a realisation that they have improved their social capital.

Further evaluation of the dimensions of social capital and how they may help explain the social position of people like George, Jenny and Janet is required.

CONCLUSION

In many ways people with intellectual disabilities still sit on the margins of society. People with intellectual disabilities are not always fully consulted as to the ways in which they may wish to be included in more mainstream activities. However, there have been unequivocal achievements made by people with intellectual disabilities themselves. The many ways in which this vulnerable group of people have strived for self advocacy is a tribute to this. A number of examples are presented within this book of where people with intellectual disabilities have influenced policy, contributed to different activities within higher education and have successfully gained employment.

This chapter has put forward a review of social inclusion and people with intellectual disabilities. It has sought to highlight the necessity of combining the two theoretical positions of social inclusion and social capital to overcome the dangers of pursuing a single concept to assess improvements in the lives of people with intellectual disabilities.

The landscape of care and delivery is changing once again for this group of people. If robust monitoring measures to guide the development of the emerging self-directed forms of care such as Direct Payments and Individual Budgets can be found, then this, as one example, holds some hope for the choice agenda. However, too much emphasis on self determined forms of care that in reality can never be properly resourced or supported presents a danger that raised expectations will not be met. Inclusive thinking in this sense equates to a dogmatic pursuit of ideology. Inclusive thinking that adopts the potential of a social capitalist perspective that is grounded in empirical evaluation, user and practice wisdom to inform that decision making, holds more substance.

The balance between protection and properly supporting choice and the promotion of rights needs to be found to adequately modernise intellectual disability care. Where such arguments are too firmly based on the persistent theoretical distinction between impairment and disability is not seen as helpful.

As the landscape of social care for people with intellectual disabilities and their carers is set to change over the next 5 years, commissioners and managers of services require further encouragement to adopt both social capital and social inclusion principles to inform their decision making. A literature that reviews both these concepts for their viability and usefulness has not yet emerged. Although the adoption of social capital and social inclusion principles are not a panacea for improving the lives of people with intellectual disability, without further evaluation of such principles, intellectual disability provision could continue to follow a path of ideology, rather than one based on empirical evaluation. More importantly, social capital is seen as essential to achieve effective citizenship (Giddens 2006:675), a key aspiration grounded within the *Valuing People* document (Department of Health 2001). Unless people with intellectual disabilities find more leverage and social control for themselves and/or those who continue to work with them continue to support them do so, the foundations to realise political inclusive statements will always be on unstable ground.

REFERENCES

Armstrong D 2002 The politics of self-advocacy and people with learning disabilities. Policy and Politics 20: 196-213.

Baron S, Field J, Schuller T 2000 Social capital: critical perspectives. Oxford University Press.

Bates P, Davies F A 2004 Social capital, social inclusion and services for people with learning disabilities. Disability and Society 19(3):195-207.

Beange H 2000 Intellectual disability and health care: the size of the problem. University of Sydney: Centre for Developmental Disability Studies.

Brown P, Lauder H, 2000 Human capital, social capital, and collective intelligence. In: Baron S,

Field S, Schuller T (eds) Social capital: critical perspectives. Oxford University Press, pp 226–242.

Bury M 1997 Health and illness in a changing society. Routledge, London.

Bury M 2000 A comment on the ICIDH2. Disability and Society 15(7):1073-1077.

Byrne D 2005 Social exclusion: issues in society. Open University Press.

Capriano R M 2007 Neighbourhood social capital and adult health: an empirical test of a bourdieu based model. Health and Place 13:639-655.

Clouston E 2008 On a roll in www.guardian.co.uk/society/2008/jan16/learning disability.

Coleman J 1988 Social capital in the creation of human capital. American Journal of Sociology 94(suppl):S99-S120.

Coleman J C 1994 Foundations of social theory. Harvard University Press, Cambridge, MA.

Department of Health Signposts for success: a guide for effective commissioning of services for people with learning disabilities. HMSO, London.

Department of Health 2000 The national health service plan. HMSO, London.

Department of Health 2001 Valuing people: a new strategy for people with learning disabilities for the 21st century. HMSO, London.

Department of Health 2005 …The story so far…Valuing people: a new strategy for learning disability for the 21st century. HMSO, London.

Department of Health 2006 Our health our say: A new direction for community services. Department of Health, London.

Department of Health 2007a Good practice in learning disability nursing. Department of Health, London.

Department of Health 2007b Progress to transformation. Department of Health, London.

Department of Health 2007c Putting people first: a shared vision and commitment to the transformation of adult social care. Department of Health, London.

Disability Rights Commission 2006 Equal treatment: closing the gap. A report into the inequalities in physical health experienced by people mental health problems and learning disabilities. Disability Rights Commission, London.

Emerson E, Hatton C 1996 Deinstitutionalization in the UK and Ireland: outcomes for service users. Journal of Intellectual Disability Research 21:17-37.

Emerson E, McVilly K 2004 Friendship activities of adults with intellectual disabilities in supported accommodation in Northern England. Journal of Applied Research in Intellectual Disabilities 17:191-197.

Fairclough N 2000 New labour, new language. Routledge, London.

Folland S 2007 Does community social capital contribute to population health? Social Science and Medicine 64:2342-2354.

General Social Care Council 2002 Codes of practice for social work. GSCC.

Giddens A 2006 Chapter 16 in Organizations and networks in sociology, 5th edn. Polity Press, Cambridge.

Halpern D 2005 Social capital. Polity Press, Cambridge.

Hancock T 2001 People, partnerships and human progress: building community capital. Health Promotion International 16(3):275-280.

Hardy S, Kramer R, Holt G et al 2006 Supporting complex needs: a practical guide for support staff working with people with a learning disability who have a mental health needs. Turning Point, London.

Isalm M K, Merlo J, Kawachi I et al 2006 Social capital and health: does egalitarianism matter? A literature review. International Journal for Equity and Health 5(3):1-28.

Labonte R 2004 Social inclusion/exclusion: dancing the dialetic. Health Promotion International 19(1):115-121.

Marshall D 2006 Positive images. Learning Disability Practice 9(6):22-23.

McConkey R 2007 Variations in the social inclusion of people with intellectual disabilities in supported living schemes and residential settings. Journal of Intellectual Disability Research 51(3):207-217.

Mencap 1999 Living in fear. Mencap, London.

Mencap 2007 Death by indifference: following up the treat me right report. Mencap, London.

Myers F, Ager A, Kerr P, Myles S 1998 Outside looking in? Studies of the community integration of people with learning disabilities. Disability and Society 13(93):389-413.

Oliver M 1996 Understanding disability: from theory to practice. Macmillan, Basingstoke.

Oxford Dictionary 1997 latest edition. Oxford University Press, Oxford.

Pavey B 2006 Human capital, social capital, entrepreneurship and disability: an examination of some current educational trends in the UK. Disability and Society 21(3):217-229.

Portes A 1998 Social capital: its origins and applications in modern sociology. Annual Review of Sociology 24:1-24.

Putnam R 1995 Bowling alone: America's declining social capital. Journal of Democracy 6.

Putnam R 2000 Bowling alone: the collapse and revival of American community. Simon & Schuster, New York.

Redley M, Weinberg D 2007 Learning disability and the limits of liberal citizenship: interactional impediments to political empowerment. Sociology of Health and Illness 29(5):767-786.

Riddell S, Baron S, Stalker K, Wilkinson H 1997 The concept of the learning society for adults with learning difficulties: human and social capital perspectives. Journal of Education Policy 12(6):473-483.

Royal College of Nursing 1980 Community Services for people with a mental handicap. RCN, London.

Shakespeare T 2006 Disability rights and wrongs. Routledge, London.

Thomas C 1999 Female forms: experiencing and understanding disability. Open University Press, Buckingham.

Thomas C 2004 Rescuing a social relational understanding of disability. Scandinavian Journal of Disability Research 6(1):22-36.

Wilkinson R G 1996 Unhealthy societies: the affliction of inequalities. Routledge, London.

Williams S J 1999 Is there anybody out there? Critical realism. Chronic illness and the disability debate. Sociology of Health and Illness 21(6):797-819.

World Health Organization 1980 International classification of impairments, disabilities and handicaps, Geneva: World Health Organization.

The legacy of 'Valuing People' in England

3

John Turnbull

INTRODUCTION

The publication in March 2001 of 'Valuing People', the Government's White Paper on learning disability (Department of Health 2001), was given a qualified welcome by people with intellectual disabilities, their relatives and staff working in services. Judging by published comments at the time the Government was applauded by many for its vision and commitment to improve life chances for people with intellectual disabilities (Turnbull 2001) but others were sceptical of its capacity to supply the resources to achieve its ambition (Beacock 2001, Foundation for People with Learning Disabilities 2001). Whatever their view on the detail of the White Paper or the many resource issues, everyone at the time seemed convinced that Valuing People would play a significant role in the years to come in the lives of people with intellectual disabilities and those who supported them (Gates 2001).

A little over 6 years since its publication this chapter aims to reflect on this viewpoint and ask what is the legacy of Valuing People in England and, more specifically, has it had the impact on people's lives that was predicted? While it might seem premature to pose such a question, it is worth acknowledging that it seems that the Government has been having similar thoughts. For example, a news report in Community Care (Taylor 2007) quoted an announcement by the Care Services Minister, Ivan Lewis, that a refresher document on intellectual disabilities would be produced by his department later in 2007 in order to add impetus to the implementation of Valuing People. The news report speculated whether there had been some disappointment within Government that targets had been missed and that Partnership Boards, introduced as part of the White Paper, had been ineffective.

This chapter will begin by briefly clarifying the status of a document such as a White Paper and reflecting on whether it is feasible for one document to have an impact, by itself, on the lives of people with intellectual disabilities and will ask what other factors might help or hinder its implementation? The remainder of the chapter will provide an overview of the emerging evidence of the impact of Valuing People on the lives of people with intellectual disabilities and the services they use.

This chapter will draw upon a range of documentary evidence from people with intellectual disabilities using the services of a NHS Trust in the south of England that provides both specialist health and social care. More specifically this information consists of the outcome of two surveys of the experiences of people with intellectual disabilities using the various short-term assessment and treatment facilities within the specialist health service directorate of the Trust. The discussion will also be informed by sections of the quarterly performance reports made to the Trust Board over a 12-month period. These reports are used routinely to inform the Trust about the impact of its health and social care services on the lives of people and the quality of its services and have been designed to complement the principles of Valuing People.

WHITE PAPERS AND SOCIAL CHANGE

In order to evaluate the impact of Valuing People there is a need to understand the context in which such documents are published and how they fit in with the overall process of social change. White Papers are published in the expectation that they will be carried out in full. White Papers don't have the force of law, though many will contain details of any new legislation that the Government needs to introduce to ensure its wishes are carried out. In the case of Valuing People no legislation was required. White Papers also typically contain details of the resources that the Government intends to make available to implement any initiatives. In Valuing People's case the Government highlighted several areas in which it intended to make resources available, for example in supporting self advocacy and in extending training opportunities for new staff in intellectual disability services.

In his preface to Valuing People the then Prime Minister, Tony Blair, stated that White Papers, by themselves, could not bring about change. This is most certainly true and the Prime Minister's comments in this instance were probably directed to the thousands of people whose efforts would be needed to turn the good intentions of the White Paper into reality. However, there are other reasons why White Papers need more than good intentions and good will to make them achieve change. Many of these reasons are practical ones. For example, as Race (2007) pointed out, it may be easier for Government strategies to be implemented in the National Health Service (NHS) because it is a national bureaucracy controlled by ministers. Local implementation becomes more difficult when Government policies and strategies have to be routed through the different layers of Local Government that exist each of which has its own elected politicians in positions of power and influence. In the case of Valuing People, Race (2007) also points out that many of its initiatives require local NHS and Local Authority to collaborate to bring about change. Where relationships between the two agencies are good, this presents few problems. However, where tensions exist, there will inevitably be in-fighting over access to and control of resources. It is impossible to quantify precisely how this has affected the implementation of Valuing People but this may account for the delay in achieving several of the targets that require multi-agency collaboration.

To anyone who has worked in the NHS or a Local Authority Race's observations are accurate but they also raise broader issues about how social change is brought about in the United Kingdom and the role played by power struggles between groups in determining what change happens, when, and for what reasons. For example, Person Centred Planning is an initiative that is championed by Valuing People but could present a challenge to some aspects of

INTELLECTUAL DISABILITY AND SOCIAL INCLUSION

professional practice whose focus is on assessment and need identification. Likewise, Valuing People raised questions about the structure and functions of Learning Disability Teams and called for them to be reviewed. This could raise anxieties among those managing and working in teams. Finally, the target for the closure of the remaining NHS-run long stay residential establishments may cause difficulties both for NHS Trusts who must transfer responsibility, and in some cases the staff, to social care providers and the Local Authority who must accept that responsibility.

Issues such as these are not exclusive to Valuing People and apply to almost any Government policy and initiative. However, they are relevant to this examination of the legacy of Valuing People because they show how critical it is to the success of White Papers that there is local change management capacity and capability as well as strong national leadership.

At a local level Valuing People introduced Partnership Boards which were intended to bring together service providers, commissioners and service users to oversee the implementation of Valuing People at a local level. Although Partnership Boards have probably brought many benefits such as encouraging multi-agency collaboration and providing opportunities to hear the voice of people with intellectual disabilities, they have suffered because they have no statutory role within the overall structure of services and decision making (Fryson & Ward 2004). When it comes to allocating resources, these are still under the control of the Local Authority and the local health commissioners. Therefore, it ought to be conceded that Partnership Boards have been a disappointing and ineffective means of bringing about change. Progress in achieving Valuing People targets may also have been delayed by the Department of Health itself. Intellectual disability is a small part of the overall work of the Department and there is a need to raise the profile of Valuing People's principles and targets and integrate them into the decision making process at both a local and national level. Unfortunately, national performance targets for the NHS and Local Authorities have not included Valuing People targets which means that there are few incentives for decision makers to drive local change (Mir 2007). Therefore, any change must be seen in the light of the organisational and cultural context in which improvement is being sought. The main objectives in Valuing People are shown in Table 3.1.

VALUING PEOPLE – IMPROVING LIVES?

Moving on from the strategic level, the obvious question about Valuing People is has it improved the lives of people with intellectual disabilities? Although the question is a simple one, it is only possible to give a qualified answer because, as Emerson et al (2005) point out, the type of information needed to judge progress against Valuing People targets is not routinely produced and published. Therefore, any judgement about the impact of Valuing People must be based primarily on the one-off studies that have been taking place since its publication, most of which will be unrepresentative of the population of people with intellectual disabilities. Many of them also do not cover all of the targets in Valuing People. For instance Emerson et al (2005) could not find information or surveys relating to the objective about improving the quality of services. Finally, it must be remembered that Valuing People is only one among

Table 3.1   Valuing People objectives and number of sub-objectives

Valuing People – main objectives	Number of sub-objectives
1. Disabled children and young people To ensure that disabled children gain maximum life chance benefits from educational opportunities, health care and social care, while living with their families or other appropriate settings in the community where their assessed needs are adequately met and reviewed.	6
2. Transition into adult life As young people with intellectual disabilities move into adulthood, to ensure continuity of care and support for the young person and their family and to provide equality of opportunity in order to enable as many disabled young people as possible to participate in education, training or employment.	2
3. More choice and control To enable people with intellectual disabilities to have as much choice and control as possible over their lives through advocacy and a person-centred approach to planning the services they need.	5
4. Supporting carers To increase the help and support carers receive from all local agencies in order to fulfil their family and caring roles effectively.	4
5. Good health To enable people with intellectual disabilities to access a health service designed around their individual needs, with fast and convenient care delivered to a consistently high standard and with additional support where necessary.	3
6. Housing To enable people with intellectual disabilities and their families to have greater choice and control over where and how they live.	3
7. Fulfilling lives To enable people with intellectual disabilities to lead full and purposeful lives within their community and to develop a range of friendships, activities and relationships.	5
8. Moving into employment To enable more people with intellectual disabilities to participate in all forms of employment wherever possible in paid work and to make a valued contribution to the world of work.	3
9. Quality To ensure that all agencies commission and provide high quality, evidence based, and continuously improving services which promote both good outcomes and best value.	5
10. Workforce and planning To ensure that social and health care staff working with people with intellectual disabilities are appropriately skilled, trained and qualified and to promote a better understanding of the needs of people with intellectual disabilities among the wider workforce.	3
11. Partnership working To promote holistic services for people with intellectual disabilities through effective partnership working between all relevant local agencies in the commissioning and delivery of services.	3

a range of initiatives and policies that have the potential to affect the lives of people with intellectual disabilities. This will be discussed again later in this chapter but it means that it may not be possible to attribute any change in the lives of people with intellectual disabilities solely to Valuing People. In spite of these difficulties, this section aims to sample the main studies of the impact of Valuing People and to supplement this information with evidence from the lives of those receiving services from a NHS Trust in the south of England.

The most extensive study of the lives of people with intellectual disabilities in recent years was carried out by Emerson et al (2005) who surveyed 3000 adults in 2004. Where people were unable to respond themselves to questions, responses were elicited from people who knew the individuals well. The study did not set out to evaluate the impact of Valuing People though many of its results can be used to shed light on its possible achievements as well as the scale of the task facing it. Some of the main findings from this study are shown in Box 3.1.

The vision set out by Valuing People is of all people with intellectual disabilities participating in society, achieving their potential, enjoying optimum health and, if necessary, using services and supports that have been specifically designed around their needs and aspirations. The reality of Emerson et al's (2005) research is in stark contrast to this.

Whereas Emerson et al (2005) did not have a specific remit to evaluate progress against Valuing People targets, the annual reports to the Department of Health from the National Director for Valuing People, Rob Greig, attempted to give a more explicit account of its impact. In his report on Valuing People in 2004 (Department of Health 2004) Rob Greig listed a number of initiatives that Government departments and the National Valuing People Support Team had been undertaking to implement Valuing People objectives. However, although the message was upbeat the report lacked any systematically derived information about the impact of the White Paper on people's lives. This was remedied to a certain extent the following year when the annual report used a range of information sources including 581 responses from people with intellectual disabilities to questions asking for their opinion on whether there had been improvements in the previous five years in areas that corresponded to

---

Box 3.1 Main findings from the study of people's lifestyles by Emerson et al (2005)

- 1 in 6 people of working age had a job
- 2 out of 3 people who were unemployed who could work said they would like a job
- 19% of people living away from their family home never saw their families
- 31% of people said they had no contact with friends
- 5% of people reported feeling extremely lonely
- 69% of people said their friends also had intellectual disabilities
- 43% of people said they had been bullied
- 32% of people said they didn't always feel safe

the Valuing People objectives (Department of Health 2005a). Overall, their responses showed that they believed that Valuing People had got better for some people but not all. The greatest area for optimism seemed to be their belief that training for staff had got better and the area of greatest disappointment seemed to come from a lack of jobs where most people thought either that things hadn't changed or had got worse. Interestingly, individuals also expressed the view that support for family carers did not seem to have changed much and people also felt that help to improve health had either not changed or only changed for some. Self advocacy groups throughout the country were also asked to contribute to the evaluation of the White Paper. Their questionnaire was different but their views were similar to those of individuals in that they believed that the situation regarding jobs for people with intellectual disabilities had not changed. The groups were equally divided on whether help for people's health had improved or not changed, with a few stating that matters had got worse. The area that most people reported had got worse was in the category of 'money'. These views are interesting in that they have been explicitly linked to Valuing People targets. However, they may not be representative of people with intellectual disabilities and their validity could also be questioned because it is unclear how much help people needed to express their opinion. Although in this report Rob Greig claimed that Valuing People was a success, the opinions of people with intellectual disabilities are not exactly ringing endorsements of the White Paper and they must be seen in the light of Emerson et al's (2005) more substantial survey. Therefore, the phrase 'cautiously optimistic' might have been more appropriate for Rob Greig to use.

Alongside his report in 2005 the National Director also published a document called 'Valuing People – what do the numbers tell us?' (Department of Health 2005b). This contained additional information that had been obtained from local authorities and the NHS on strategic level change, some of which Rob Greig admitted could not be verified. Despite this, the brief report shows a mixed picture of change. Among the good news is that there had been an increase in the amount of people with intellectual disabilities receiving direct payments. More people are receiving short breaks, fewer people were living in NHS long stay accommodation and that the amount of spending on advocacy had increased from £60 per person in 2001 to stand at £140 per person in 2004/05. Amongst the disappointing news was the fact that only one in ten people with intellectual disabilities had a job and that people from different ethnic backgrounds appeared not to be accessing services. In his report Greig raises the issue of a lack of routinely collected information which has made it difficult to assess the impact of Valuing People. Added to this is the fact that much of the information cited related to inputs and processes connected to the lives of people with intellectual disabilities and the services they use but little is revealed about their impact on people's lifestyles.

The Emerson et al (2005) survey and the 2005 annual report on Valuing People from Rob Greig have taken a broad view of the lives of people with intellectual disabilities but it is worth noting that there have been more focused studies that have explored some of the specific objectives of Valuing People. For example, one of the key objectives of Valuing People was to encourage the development of Person Centred Planning with people with intellectual disabilities. Research by Robertson et al (2006) is probably the most extensive study of the effectiveness of Person Centred Planning as well as the costs of its implementation. The researchers spent two years following the progress of 65 people who were involved in developing their Person Centred Plan. Briefly, the findings were that there had been modest improvements in the participants' social networks, contact with their families, community activity, choice and day activities.

It is interesting to contemplate why Person Centred Planning seems to have been successful when other objectives within Valuing People have yet to be achieved. For example, Mir (2007) investigated progress against the health targets in Valuing People and concluded that only slow progress had been made. As far as Person Centred Planning was concerned, one of the possible reasons is that the Department of Health was quick to publish supplementary guidance and good practice to the publication of the White Paper itself, thus giving staff the tools to carry out their roles more easily. However, this was also true for Health Action Planning which Mir reports has been a target that has been missed. In spite of some fears that Person Centred Planning could challenge traditional professional practice, another reason for its success is the fact that it can be implemented relatively efficiently and effectively compared to other Valuing People objectives such as getting more people into work. For example, Robertson et al's (2006) research estimated that the cost of person centred plans was approximately £600 per person but that these costs would diminish over time as competency among staff was built up. This contrasts with the experience of those trying to develop Health Action Plans which Mir claims is a complex process that involves enlisting the support of general practitioners and other professionals. She also points out that there are no incentives in the system to develop Health Action Plans. Mir argues for better leadership to ensure that Health Action Planning can be co-ordinated more efficiently at a local level. Mir's experience also contrasts with that of people introducing Person Centred Plans in that Health Action Plans are a new phenomenon whereas, as Roberston et al (2006) point out, Person Centred Planning is the latest attempt by staff and others to develop a truly individualised planning system for people. Therefore, the success of Person Centred Planning should not be attributed solely to the White Paper because staff may simply be building on existing competence in planning with people.

THE VALUING PEOPLE LEGACY: A LOCAL PERSPECTIVE

As well as national initiatives that have taken place to evaluate the impact of Valuing People, providers of services to people with intellectual disabilities have also been interested in monitoring their own progress against the principles and targets of the White Paper. A specialist NHS Trust in the south of England takes a variety of approaches to achieve this and some of the measures will now be described.

The Trust provides a range of short term residential services for people who have severe challenging behaviour who need assessment and treatment, for people who have severe challenging behaviour and mental health problem as well as a forensic service.

Two years ago the service initiated an annual survey of people living in these facilities in order to learn how people were living their lives, what they thought about the quality of their support and whether the principles and some of the targets in Valuing People were being adhered to. Participation in the survey was entirely voluntary and responses were treated in confidence. Each person was interviewed by a trained interviewer who was someone who did not work in the particular facility. It is only possible to provide a snapshot of responses and comments but full copies of the survey results can be obtained from the author.

In the 2005 survey 48 people were approached to take part and 30 agreed. Two thirds of people said they always felt listened to by staff and were supported to make choices and the other third said they felt listened to and supported sometimes.

> 'The OT team are good here... I trust some people who work here but others I don't trust'

> 'People listen to me'

Most people said that they had their treatment and medication explained to them and all but one person reported that they had received help to stay healthy. All of the service users had a care plan but it was disappointing that only half reported that they had been involved in developing their plan or had copies of it. It is possible that some of those responding to the survey were relative newcomers who had yet to be involved in developing their plan further. Of those who reported having been involved, they also reported that their friends and relatives had been included. In terms of their day-to-day lives most people reported that they had regular contact with the community and had been out and about though some people clearly did not think this sufficient. These activities consisted mainly of shopping, visiting relatives, walking in the countryside.

> 'My care team take me out on nice days shopping for new clothes'

> 'I would like more walks'

> 'I would like to go out more and join in with things outside the unit like try working or maybe going to college'

Three people described the help they had received finding work and two of them obtained work whilst living in the Trust's facilities. Finally, a third of respondents said they knew about local self-advocacy services.

The following year's survey showed similar results but only 25 people took part. People still felt listened to though some felt very strongly that they were not understood.

> 'People listen to me... me and my team are going to teach other staff and service users how to use Makaton.'

> 'I wasn't listened to when I first arrived and staff did not know what my diagnosis was. I wish that staff would find out more about my problems to ease my distress as I feel I'm getting worse.'

The exceptions were a reported increase in the support people received to go out of the facilities and engage in activities in the community.

> 'I like it when staff take me for picnics, pub lunches and boat rides'

> 'I like discos and the buffet foods at discos'

There had also been a dramatic increase in the provision of advocacy services which resulted in just over half the people reporting that they had an independent advocate. People also reported having greater access to 'talking therapies'. The level of involvement in personal planning was about the same as reported previously.

Elsewhere in the Trust, performance information is routinely collected and published on the services provided to over two hundred people who are living in supported living arrangements. This information is initially presented in the form of a quarterly performance reports to the Trust Board. However, each quarter a Valuing People theme is chosen and reported on in greater depth. The current system was redeveloped in 2004 to incorporate Valuing People themes. Three quarterly reports were chosen at random to summarise for the purposes of this chapter. The report from March 2007 focused on choice and asked a range of questions of service users and staff about choices made about their living arrangements. 56% of people said they were involved in choosing the people who support them. 51% of people said they had people involved in their support other than paid staff which is part of the aims of the service to vary the interaction and relationships engaged in by service users. On the other hand, 52% of people reported that they had no choice over whom they live with but over half of these respondents said they were happy with the arrangements. These responses are slightly better than those reported in some of the national surveys referred to earlier but it must be remembered that these figures are unrepresentative.

In June 2006, the quarterly report focused on Person Centred Planning. All respondents were found to have Person Centred Plans and 55% of plans were rated as being completely reflective of the individual and their needs and wishes. Those involved in the rating exercise evaluated 35% of plans as being reflective of most aspects of the individual. The ratings also concluded that the support provided was organised mostly in line with the Person Centred Plan. It was also found that only 3% of plans had not been reviewed. These figures suggest that the Trust has been both efficient and effective in fulfilling the aim in Valuing People relating to Person Centred Planning.

The theme for the report in December 2005 was partnership and explored all aspects of partnership both between the Trust and service users and relatives as well as the Trust and other providers. The staff and managers in the service could point to a great deal of evidence to demonstrate how well they were working with other providers which resulted in them being given an 'excellent' or 'good' rating. In contrast relationships with families in 15–20% of areas was rated as poor. Another aspect of good news was that relationships between the tenants in the houses and their registered social landlord was rated as positive with many examples of tenants participating in tenants groups.

SO, WHAT IS THE LEGACY OF VALUING PEOPLE?

This concluding section will aim to bring together the key issues arising out of the implementation of Valuing People in order to arrive at a view on the nature of the legacy of Valuing People in England. The evidence on how people with intellectual disabilities are leading their lives suggests a varied position in that some people may have improved their lives and there may have been improvements in some aspects of most people's lives. Although overall progress may be slow, the greatest progress seems to have been made in the development of Person Centred Planning and the area in which there seems to have been no improvement is that of developing work opportunities for people with intellectual disabilities. There is a suggestion within the literature that change may be more difficult for some groups within the population of people with intellectual disabilities. For example, people from different ethnic backgrounds do not appear to be accessing services and appear to be worse off on most of the lifestyle indicators within the studies discussed above. People who are undergoing or about to undergo a transition in their lives whether from childhood into adulthood or into old age also seem unprepared for this change. People with high support needs also seem more likely to have fewer choices and lead more isolated lives. Obviously it is difficult to be definitive about attributing any change to Valuing People because information on lifestyles was not routinely collected prior to its publication. However, these are two groups for whom the planners, managers and staff working in the field of intellectual disability will need to invest further resources to prevent them becoming even more isolated and left behind if the pace of change increases.

On the issue of resources, the process of implementing Valuing People so far has provided some interesting instruction for people working to bring about change. For example Robertson et al (2006) showed that Person Centred Planning and improvements associated with it could be introduced with relatively little investment which would reduce as staff competence increased. Its success could probably be attributed to the fact that Person Centred Planning builds on previous knowledge, it is dependent largely upon existing staff working in the field of intellectual disability, it has some immediate 'products' in the form of plans which, in turn, present opportunities for services to measure progress. Elsewhere the lessons seem harder to learn, especially where multi-agency collaboration is required or where the support of people outside of the intellectual disability service community is needed. Here, the legacy of Valuing People seems to be that insufficient investment was made in creating incentives for change. As Rob Greig points out poignantly in his report to the Department of Health in 2005:

> 'In some other places, little has changed. Put bluntly, too many people in public services see Valuing People as being 'optional' – something they can get away with not doing.'
>
> Department of Health 2005

Perhaps the promised review of Valuing People (Taylor 2007) will give the Government the opportunity to put more incentives for change in place. It would also be wise to revisit the way in which its objectives were written. For example, it could be that one of the reasons why there are few incentives to implement change is that the objectives are too broad and do not lend themselves easily to measurement and monitoring by relevant organisations.

If some people in organisations have found it difficult to become enthusiastic about Valuing People, one of the legacies of the White Paper must be that it has generated interest and commitment from many working within intellectual disability services. It is now difficult to imagine a situation before Valuing People came along. However, there was a feeling that most of the relics of a previous era had been removed from the landscape such as long stay hospitals but that something else was needed to fill the void. Valuing People certainly helped to re-energise and refresh the thinking of those working with people with intellectual disabilities. Whether it has completely filled the gap is doubtful. It may ultimately prove that other elements that are part of the Government's social inclusion agenda will be more effective at bringing about change. For example, the Disability Discrimination Act and Human Rights Act may be more powerful in improving lifestyles by reminding people of their responsibilities and enabling excluded people to access their rights. Likewise, within services, the Cornwall Report (Commission for Health Improvement and Commission for Social Care Inspection 2006) and 'Death by Indifference' (2007) have probably been more effective than Valuing People in generating action. This serves as a useful reminder that Valuing People is part of a wider process of social change and that not everything related to intellectual disability began with its publication. Nevertheless, it will continue to be a prominent signpost in the journey towards inclusion and improved life chances for people with intellectual disabilities.

REFERENCES

Beacock C 2001 Counting the cost. Learning Disability Practice 4(1):5.

Department of Health 2001 Valuing People. A new strategy for learning disability for the 21st century. Department of Health, London.

Department of Health 2004 The Government's annual report on learning disability 2004. Valuing People: moving forward together. Department of Health, London.

Department of Health 2005a The government's annual report on learning disability 2005. Department of Health, London.

Department of Health 2005b Valuing People – what do the numbers tell us? Department of Health, London.

Emerson E, Malam S, Davies I, Spencer K 2005 Adults with Learning Difficulties in England 2003/04. Office of National Statistics, London.

Foundation for People with Learning Disabilities 2001 Great White Paper but is there money to implement it? News Release, 23rd March 2001. Foundation for People with Learning Disabilities, London.

Fryson R, Ward L 2004 Making Valuing People work: strategies for change in services for people with learning disabilities. Policy Press, Bristol.

Gates B 2001 Valuing People. Editorial. Journal of Learning Disabilities 5(3):203-207.

Healthcare Commission and Commission for Social Care Inspection 2006 Joint investigation into the provision of services for people with learning disabilities at Cornwall Partnership NHS Trust, London. HCC/CSCI.

MENCAP 2007 Death by Indifference. MENCAP, London.

Mir G 2007 Meeting Valuing People health targets: recommendations from a research workshop. British Journal of Learning Disabilities 35(2):75-83.

Race D 2007 A tale of two White Papers: policy documents as indicators of trends in UK services. Journal of Intellectual Disabilties 11(1):83-103.

Roberston J, Emerson E, Hatton C et al 2006 Longitudinal analysis of the impact and cost of person centred planning for people with intellectual disabilities in England. American Journal on Mental Retardation 111(6):400-416.

Taylor A 2007 Minister: we're struggling with Valuing People goals. Community Care. 3rd May 2001. pp 7.

Turnbull J 2001 Lead on. Learning Disability Practice 4(1):2.

LIVERPOOL JOHN MOORES UNIVERSITY
LEARNING SERVICES

Policy in Scotland: implementing 'The same as you?'

Michael Brown

4

INTRODUCTION

This chapter will detail Scottish policy and the developments that have resulted since political devolution and the publication of *The same as you?* by the government in 2000. An analysis of the involvement of people with intellectual disabilities as users of public services will be explored and their part in the policy process and the impact of *The same as you?* on their lives.

There is an evolving and developing body of literature relating to the place of people with intellectual disabilities in the research process. Little however has been written about their contribution and involvement within the policy process. This is a significant gap and is an area requiring further investigation and enquiry. This chapter seeks to begin to address this gap by examining the contributions made by people with intellectual disabilities throughout the policy process and identify what they think has been achieved as a result.

Two Directors from People First Scotland, a key national self advocacy organisation comprising people with intellectual disabilities, participated in semi-structured policy-focused interviews. During the interviews they detailed their involvement in developing policy and influencing and supporting the implementation of policy intended to improve the lives of people with intellectual disabilities in Scotland.

THEORIES, MODELS AND THE POLICY PROCESS

Critical Social Theory is a model that has attracted attention in intellectual disability practice due to the focus on issues of oppression of minority groups and the distribution of power and resources within society (Munhall 2007, Owen-Mills 1995). As a model, Critical Social Theory seeks to enable action and change that is transformational and in the case of people with intellectual disabilities, challenge their exclusion and marginalisation as equal citizens (Gilbert 2004, Walmsley 2001).

There is now increasing recognition of the need to develop and increase the research evidence-base in intellectual disabilities (Barr 2007). Despite the recognition, significant challenges exist in undertaking research that adds to and evolves the evidence-base and is also inclusive of people with intellectual disabilities (NHS Health Scotland 2004, Brown 2007). One area that has attracted interest in an attempt to address these issues are the emancipatory and participatory research paradigms that aims to include people with intellectual disabilities as partners and collaborators within the research process (Chappell 2000, Northway 2000a, Richardson 2000, Walmsley 2004). By adopting such approaches the stereotype of people with intellectual disabilities as oppressed and powerless is challenged (Northway 1997). From a research perspective Northway (2000b) refers to the concept of people with intellectual disabilities as research partners, while Walmsley (2004b) uses the term inclusive research to describe the roles and responsibilities adopted in the process. While there is an evolving focus on the involvement of people with intellectual disabilities in research, there has been less attention on their role within the policy process.

Policy and the policy process is essentially concerned with who gets what, when they get it and how they get it within democratic political processes (Hill 2005). At the heart of the policy process is the concept of power; and the dominant influence will focus on who has it and how it is used to influence and make decisions (Buse et al 2005). It is also important to consider and identify the reasons why an issue becomes a specific focus for policy that then requires attention. The question of how the policy area became an issue and who had the power and influence to get it there requires to be considered. The stated intentions behind the policy focus, the resources available for the delivery of the policy and the anticipated policy impacts are central to influencing the overall outcomes (Peckham & Meerabeau 2007). Closely linked to policy intent is the interface between research generated evidence and the impact of policy is important according to Lowes & Hulatt (2005).

If for example the overall stated intention of a policy initiative is to improve the lives of people with intellectual disabilities, ensuring they are involved in and throughout the policy process seems reasonable. By adopting what is termed a 'bottom-up' rather than a 'top-down' approach, the users of services can become key actors in the policy process. This places the users of services at the centre of the policy process, as the policy outcomes are intended to and will impact significantly on their lives (Hill & Hupe 2002). Collectively these issues influence and shape how users of services are engaged within the policy process.

True involvement extends beyond merely inviting participation in satisfaction surveys and questionnaires, however there is no 'right' way to involve people who use services. There are principles of effective user involvement in the policy process that have been identified. The principles include identifying the support that enables them to get together to be involved, ensuring equal opportunities for involvement exists and equal access to participate throughout all aspects of the policy process. Arising from these issues is the need to consider and take account of the needs of possible vulnerable groups, such as those with intellectual disabilities and dementia as well as potential ethical issues (Lowes & Hulatt 2005).

DEVOLUTION AND THE POLICY CONTEXT IN SCOTLAND

Government devolution took place in Scotland in 1999 and, as a result, a range of policy areas are devolved issues for the Scottish government. Key policy areas such as health and social care services are examples of such devolved policy areas, bringing about a divergence of the policy focus and priorities. There has been a significant focus on the needs of children and adults with intellectual disabilities since devolution that has resulted in a distinctly Scottish approach to services. In May 2000 the Scottish Executive published *The same as you? A review of services for people with learning disabilities in Scotland* (Scottish Executive 2000). There has been a similar focus on developing policy on the needs of people with intellectual disabilities in England, Northern Ireland and Wales (Department of Health 2001, Welsh Assembly 2002, Department of Health, Social Services and Public Safety 2004).

There has been a specific focus on the contributions required from all nurses and midwives in Scotland to contribute to addressing the health inequalities experienced by people with intellectual disabilities (Scottish Executive 2002). The issue of health needs and health inequalities was analysed by NHS Health Scotland, Scotland's national health improvement organisation, who published two major pieces of work detailing the action necessary to address the needs of people on the autism spectrum and children and adults with intellectual disabilities (Public Health Institute 2001, NHS Health Scotland 2004). The Scottish Intercollegiate Guidelines Network (SIGN) published clinical guidelines by way of *The Assessment, diagnosis and clinical interventions for children and young people with autism spectrum disorders* to assist professionals and improve clinical care for this group (SIGN 2007).

The Scottish review set out and established the policy of services providing care and support for children and adults with intellectual disabilities. Set around seven principles that make explicit the value-base that should inform and direct all services received by this group, the report states that people with intellectual disabilities should be:

- Valued
- Treated as individuals
- Asked about what they need and should be involved in making choices.
- Given the help and support to do what they want to do.
- Able to get local services like everyone else.
- Able to get specialist services when they need them.
- Able to have services that take account of their age, abilities and needs.

Twenty-nine recommendations (Box 4.1) set out the actions to be undertaken over a 10-year period to achieve the aspirations set out within the report.

Developments arising from the implementation of *The same as you?*

The recommendations contained within *The same as you?* are being implemented by a national implementation group and a range of developments have taken place since 2000. *The same as you?* requires partnership working between local authorities, NHS boards, the independent sector and people with intellectual disabilities and their families to bring about implementation. As a result, people with intellectual disabilities and their carers have been at the heart of the initiatives.

Box 4.1   Overview of the recommendations in *The same as you?*

- The developing partnership-in-practice agreements between local authorities and NHS boards
- A government change fund to support local service developments
- The developing local advocacy
- The closure of all long-stay institutions by 2005
- The development of NHS boards providing four assessment and treatment units of four beds per hundred thousand population
- The development of NHS board community services to avoid unnecessary hospital admission
- The development of support services for people with challenging behaviours
- The development of local area co-ordination to provide local support and advice

- The establishment of the Scottish Consortium for Learning Disability
- A long-term programme to raise public awareness of intellectual disabilities
- A Scottish Service Network for autism
- The development of life-long plans for those that want them
- Direct payments made available by 2003 for those who want them
- The commissioning of research focusing on people with intellectual disabilities in secure environments
- The training for professionals to enable identification of dementia
- Undertake a national review of speech and language therapy requirements

THE SCOTTISH CONSORTIUM FOR LEARNING DISABILITY

The Scottish Consortium for Learning Disability (SCLD) came about from Recommendation 6 of *The same as you?*, which stated that:

> 'The Scottish Executive should set up a new Scottish centre for learning disability. This would offer advice, training and support to agencies, professionals, people with learning disabilities and parents to bring about the changes we have recommended in this review.'
>
> Scottish Executive 2000:26

SCLD was established October 2001 to offer support to implement *The same as you?* by enabling the development of services to promote collaboration, disseminate research findings that improve lives. SCLD is made up of 13 partner organisations that have joined together with funding from the Scottish Executive to become the Scottish Consortium for Learning Disability. The 13 partners are ARC Scotland, Badaguish Outdoor Centre, 'BILD' British Institute of Learning Disabilities, Capability Scotland, Key Housing Association, PAMIS, Quality Action Group, the University of Abertay – The Tayside Institute of Health Studies, University of Dundee – The White Top Research Unit, which conducts multidisciplinary research in the area of profound and multiple disability, the University of St Andrews and the Glasgow University Affiliated Programme comprising a number of departments with interests in people with intellectual disabilities including:

- The Department of Psychological Medicine
- The Strathclyde Centre for Disability Research
- The Nuffield Centre for Community Care Studies
- The Department of Educational Studies
- The Department of General Practice

SCLD have been remitted with key areas to support the implementation of *The same as you?* One of the key functions is to develop and improve training and education across sectors. Another is to support the development of a national network for people with profound and multiple impairment which has been established in collaboration with PAMIS (Promoting A More Inclusive Society), one of the SCLD partner organisations. SCLD have also developed a national campaign, *Changing Hearts and Minds*, which supports *The same as you?* recommendation that seeks to change public attitudes towards people with intellectual disabilities in their communities.

The 2000 review stated that local databases for people with learning disabilities and their needs should be developed. This has led to the establishment of the national eSAY project, part of the government's eCare Framework that will enable multi-agency information sharing within the public sector in Scotland (Scottish Executive 2000). eSAY is a dataset that can be used by all local authorities and health boards to collect key information in the same way that can be used to plan and develop services.

LOCAL AREA CO-ORDINATION

Local Area Co-ordination was introduced to Scotland and developed from a model found in Western Australia. With a strong, person centred value base, Local Area Co-ordination is a model that supports individuals and families to build a 'good life' and to strengthen the capacity of communities to include disabled people. To support the model, Local Area Co-ordinators (LACs), drawn from a diverse range of backgrounds, co-ordinate services, provide information about local services and support families and people with intellectual disabilities. The LACs work with a small number of people and their families to support them through the complex care systems. LACs have also been given the role of ensuring that those who want a personal life plan are supported to have one.

Research was commissioned by the government in 2006 to determine how Local Area Co-ordination is working (Scottish Executive 2007). The research found that there were 59 LACs, with most local authorities having at least one in post. Seven of the 32 local authorities in Scotland reported they did not have LACs, despite national guidance on establishing the posts. All the LACs reported working with adults and some also work with children with intellectual disabilities.

Participants in the research thought their lives were improved with LACs and they had more help regarding where to get support. However, significant variations were reported in the how LAC roles have been taken forward and this resulted in other professionals being unclear about the role. An important area of work of the LACs was in working with community groups and this was identified as an area for future development.

COMMUNITY-BASED HEALTH SERVICES

A significant recommendation related to the closure of all long stay hospitals by 2005. While significant progress has been made the government revised the target to the end of 2007 to ensure appropriate comprehensive packages of care were in place. As a result of the changes, hospitals will no longer be home for people with intellectual disabilities.

One of the principles upon which *The same as you?* is built states that those with complex needs should receive specialist service provision when necessary. From a specialist healthcare perspective this is important as the research evidence-base clearly points to the different health pattern and health needs of some people with intellectual disabilities (NHS Health Scotland 2004, Cooper et al 2004, Whitaker & Read 2006). The focus of specialist health care is predominantly community-based services and, across Scotland, Community Learning Disability Teams provide specialist domiciliary assessment, treatment, interventions for people with learning disabilities, their carers as well as support for other organisations such as general health services, social care services and the independent sector providers. In recognition of the different health needs of some people with intellectual disabilities inpatient assessment and treatment services are available and *The same as you?* recommends four beds per hundred thousand population, equating to some 400 beds across Scotland.

EVALUATING PROGRESS AND DEVELOPMENTS

To share the outcomes and developments that have taken place since the publication of *The same as you?* the government have undertaken a series of 5-year-on follow-up reports to identify developments and areas still requiring change.

Following the publication of the *Autism spectrum disorders needs assessment report*, The Same as You Implementation Group established a Scotland-wide reference group in 2002 to support the implementation of the recommendations (Public Health Institute of Scotland 2001). A number of developments have taken place and an update report was produced that sets out the achievements and areas that still require to be improved (Scottish Executive 2006d).

Home at Last? The Report on Hospital Closure Service Reprovision Sub Group – The Same As You? was published in 2003 and details the issues that required to be addressed to bring about the closure of the remaining long-stay hospital beds across Scotland (Scottish Executive 2003). The report highlights the steady decline over the past 30 years in the number of long-stay beds and the move towards community-based services. Now for those with more complex care needs, accommodation is provided in care home settings and responsibility for standards, inspection and regulation rests with the Care Commission.

Having your say? The follow up report to The same as you? review of services for people with learning disabilities – report on advocacy (Scottish Executive 2006a). This report sets out a number of action points for improving the quality and accessibility of advocacy to people of all ages, with intellectual disabilities and with autism spectrum disorders in Scotland and highlights for example that people with intellectual disabilities have a right to independent advocacy under the Mental Health (Care and Treatment) (Scotland) Act 2003.

Follow up report of The same as you? review of services for people with learning disabilities – report on children's services was published by the government and details the developments that have taken place and challenges that exist in improving the lives of children and young people with intellectual disabilities (Scottish Executive 2006b).

A follow up report of The same as you? review of services for people with learning disabilities – report on day services was published in 2006 (Scottish Executive 2006c). The report details development and changes in day services across Scotland since the publication of *The same as you?* People with intellectual disabilities and their carers were involved in the review along with local authorities and day service staff. The report highlighted the need to provide development opportunities for day service staff and to retain good workers. People with intellectual disabilities viewed employment as important and wanted further help and support to achieve this. Transport issues were reported to be a problem in some areas of Scotland and could act as a barrier to community participation for some. Family carers highlighted the need for them to be involved in decisions and development that impacted on the life of their family member.

PEOPLE FIRST SCOTLAND AND THE SAME AS YOU?

People First Scotland is a charity comprising members with an intellectual disability. The organisation is involved in a range of activities that include self advocacy, public education, campaigning for better rights, contributing to policy issues, supporting local groups of people with intellectual disabilities and providing training and support advisors. The activities of the organisation are co-ordinated by members and a Board of Directors. All the Directors are people with intellectual disabilities who are elected from geographical areas across Scotland for a period of 3 years.

Two Board Directors from *People First*, James and Steven, were interviewed to identify their views on their involvement in the development of *The same as you?* and the subsequent implementation of the recommendations. An interview schedule was developed to provide focus and structure. This was shared with James and Steven and their supporters in advance of the interview to allow them to reflect and prepare their answers. The interview was recorded and then transcribed to allow for the analysis of the data provided. The interview schedule was not prescriptive. The questions in the interview schedule can be clustered around the following headings, thereby providing structure:

- Informing and influencing policy development
- Supporting and influencing the implementation of policy
- Getting involved in policy development and implementation.

Informing and influencing the development of policy

People First members have been involved in the development of government policy and as a result have built up their knowledge and expertise. *People First* have been involved in the development of *The same as you?*, *Promoting Health, Supporting Inclusion and Promoting Access to Healthcare* (Scottish Executive 2000, 2002, and NHS Quality Improvement Scotland 2006). Following the publication of *The same as you?*, *People First* became members of the national implementation group. Their involvement demonstrates how *People First* representatives have been central to the formation and implementation of policy that directly impacts on their lives.

Steven and James believe there are a number of ways that *People First* can influence and change things for the benefit of the members. They have developed experience on a number of fronts:

- Raising awareness of the needs and view of people with intellectual disabilities nationally and locally
- Challenging situations that they believe are not right
- Talk about the things that are important to the members thereby helping others to think about people with intellectual disabilities and their needs
- Speak confidently about their needs to help others see people with intellectual disabilities as individuals

When asked about the challenges involved in getting their messages across and heard, Steven described the situation.

> 'We have to try. We have to do our best. I enjoy the challenge of getting the opinions across to officials, representatives in parliament or senior officials to listen. If you can convince the ones with the power then I think you're half way there.'
>
> Steven, Director *People First*

James described a number of ways that *People First* has tried to influence and inform decisions:

- Write letters to officials in power to highlight areas of concern and express an opinion
- Set up a meeting with officials in power to discuss issue of concern
- Lobby members of parliament to make sure they understand the needs of people with intellectual disabilities
- Challenges decisions and when things go wrong to make sure they do not happen again

Supporting and influencing the implementation of policy

Both Steven and James believe that obtaining the views and experiences of their members is vital to enable them to contribute effectively in the policy process. *People First* is organised and structured to encourage the contributions of the groups across Scotland. Local *People First* groups debate and discuss issues of concern to them and also policy issues that require the views of their members. The model is seen as central to enabling the *People First* Directors to speak for and represent the wider membership and Steven and James view representing the wider membership as an important responsibility. The views and opinions of the members of the local groups are shared with the *People First* Directors who in turn represent the wider membership. Members are according to Steven and James vocal in sharing and expressing their views. They believe the power and solidarity that can be achieved by *People First* as a collective group is considerable and there is the possibility to effect positive change for people with intellectual disabilities.

The Board of Directors of *People First* make decisions and identify their priorities from the information and views of the local groups. This is an example of a bottom-up approach, up to the wider organisation and then communicating decisions and outcomes back to the members in the local groups. The priorities set by *People First* are seen as fundamental in directing the Board of Directors.

Getting involved in policy development and implementation

James and Steven have been involved for nearly a decade in the development and implementation of *The same as you?* and both are members of the National Implementation Group. As a result of their experiences they have a wealth of knowledge to draw on and share regarding the needs and issues of concern to people with intellectual disabilities. By using the *People First* networks and structures it is possible for them to confidently represent the experiences of the members of the organisation, thereby adding credibility to their contribution within the policy process.

People with intellectual disabilities have been involved in aspects of policy over many years. Steven first became involved with *People First* over 12 years ago and has contributed to policy initiatives such as the national group supporting the implementation of *The same as you?* the 21st Century review of Social Work and Multiagency inspection programmes.

'I think I wanted to get involved because I wanted to see if I could make a difference to other people with disabilities'

Steven, Director *People First*

In order to be able to be fully involved effectively in policy initiatives, Steven and James recognise that support is seen as vital. This is provided on two fronts. *People First* supporters worked with Seven and James outwith and at formal meetings. This took the form of meeting before the 'formal' meetings to discuss the minutes from the last meeting and the agenda for the forthcoming meeting. Additionally the civil servants responsible for supporting and over viewing the implementation of *The same as you?* also offer support for James, Steven and others by ensuring minutes and other papers are produced in easy read formats. A pre meeting prior to the meeting of the main group is also held with *People First* and civil servants to discuss and identify the previous meeting and identify specific issues they might wish to raise. Steven views the support at meetings as vital to avoid him 'getting lost and losing his place' as the papers and the amount of information provided can be detailed and complex. Recognising and taking account of the additional support needs was also viewed as crucial to enable members of *People First* to contribute fully and impact effectively.

When invited to comment on the areas that Steven and James believed had made the biggest impact, Local Area Coordination was seen as important and they described their involvement in the development of the role and how they helped establish a short-life working group to oversee the work. In order for this to be successful they both recognised the additional support they required and obtained this from *People First* supporters. As representatives of members on the national implementation group, Steven and James view their priorities as to influence policy development and implementation regarding how people with intellectual disabilities live their lives in the community and what they want their lives to be. James described the situation like this:

> 'Some people are not treated very good and some are treated really poor. We want to help change that.'
>
> James, Director *People First*

People First have influenced and informed national policy implementation on a number of key fronts:

- The long-stay hospital closure programme
- Better support for parents with intellectual disabilities thereby aiming to stop their children being received into care
- Recognising the right of people with intellectual disabilities to have a relationship and sex if that is what they want

> 'Being a member of local and national implementation groups is important as we have a voice. Without that there is nothing.'
>
> Steven, Director *People First*

The same as you? said a lot about issues such as employment, housing and how money can be used to enable people with intellectual disabilities to lead independent lives. While much has been achieved as a result of their involvement in policy development and implementation, Steven and James appreciate there is still much to be done. They believe there is not enough appropriate housing and that while there has been developments in employment opportunities for some, it is harder for others with higher needs and this needs to be addressed in the future. They would also like to undertake some work on how the state benefit system can work better for people with intellectual disabilities trying to get into employment. They think this might be a barrier to preventing some moving into employment. Steven and James also want to see a continued focus on changing the views and perceptions of the general public of people with intellectual disabilities. They think this needs to start at an early age and should include further education and development opportunities for children, young people and their teachers.

Both Steven and James want to see more people with intellectual disabilities get involved in initiating, developing and implementing policies that can improve their lives as equal citizens. They would encourage others to get involved in local groups as their first step and begin to share their views and experiences. Steven summoned up his involvement like this:

> 'Well, it's quite simple, if you feel something is important, you need to get involved and try and make a difference.'
>
> Steven, Director *People First*

INTELLECTUAL DISABILITY AND SOCIAL INCLUSION

CONCLUSION

Political devolution has resulted in a policy focus on addressing the needs of people with intellectual disabilities. In Scotland there is a clear emphasis on social justice and inclusion and as a result policy makers have made significant attempts to involve people with intellectual disabilities throughout the policy process as key stakeholders. Their involvement is crucial when considered within the context of the Critical Social Theory model and the attempt to redress the power imbalance experienced by disadvantaged groups within society. Despite the attempts to include them within the policy process there is little published evidence of how people with intellectual disabilities are involved throughout the policy process and this is an area requiring further investigation and analysis. This work is necessary to help identify what has worked well and areas where further consideration and development are required.

Steven and James have developed their skills and abilities over many years in contributing to developing and implementing policy. This requires additional support from government officials and from their own organisation to enable them to contribute fully and equally. Both are independent and capable of developing their thoughts and arguments. Further consideration needs to be given to those with more complex communication needs and how their thoughts and contributions can be heard and included.

People with intellectual disabilities are capable of developing their positions on particular issues and contributing to policies aimed at improving their lives, yet they are not a homogeneous group and consideration is necessary to identify the forms of additional support required that enables them to effectively contribute. The issue of developing the capacity and capability of more people with intellectual disabilities to become involved throughout the policy process is important if their views and experiences are to be fully incorporated in the future.

Policy in Scotland

REFERENCES

Barr O 2007 Research in learning disability nursing: importance and relevance to all areas of nursing. Journal of Research in Nursing 12:107-109.

Brown M 2007 Conducting focus groups with people with learning disabilities: theoretical and practical issues. Journal of Research in Nursing 12:127-128.

Buse K, Mays N, Walt G 2005 Making health policy. Open University Press, Maidenhead.

Chappell A 2000 Emergence of participatory methodology in learning difficulty research: Understanding the context. British Journal of Learning Disabilities 28:38-43.

Cooper S-A, Melville C, Morrison J 2004 People with intellectual disabilities: Their health needs differ and need to be recognised and met. British Medical Journal 239:414-415.

Department of Health 2001 Valuing People: a new strategy for learning disability for the 21st Century. HMSO, London.

Department of Health, Social Services and Public Safety 2004 Equal Lives: Review of Policy and Services for People with Learning Disabilities in Northern Ireland. Stormont, Belfast.

Gilbert T 2004 Involving people with learning disabilities in research: issues and possibilities. Health and Social Care in the Community 12(4):298-308.

Hill M 2005 The public policy process. Pearson Longman, Essex.

Hill M, Hupe P 2002 Implementing public policy. Sage, London.

Lowes L, Hulatt I 2005 Involving service users in health and social care research. Routledge, Oxfordshire.

Munhall P 2007 Nursing research: A qualitative perspective. Jones & Bartlett, London.

NHS Health Scotland 2004 People with learning disabilities in Scotland: The Health Needs Assessment Report. Glasgow: NHS Health Scotland.

NHS Quality Improvement Scotland 2006 Promoting Access to Healthcare for people with learning disabilities. NHS Quality Improvement Scotland, Edinburgh.

Northway R 1997 Disability and oppression: Some implications for nurses and nursing. Journal of Advanced Nursing 28:736-743.

Northway R 2000a Disability, nursing research and the importance of reflexivity. Journal of Advanced Nursing 32:391-397.

Northway R 2000b The relevance of participatory research in developing nursing research and practice. Nursing Researcher 7(4):40-52.

Owen-Mills V 1995 A synthesis of praxis and critical social theory in an emancipatory curriculum. Journal of Advanced Nursing 21(6):1191-1195.

Peckham S, Meerabeau L 2007 Social policy for nurses and the helping professions. Open University Press, Maidenhead.

Public Health Institute of Scotland 2001 Autistic spectrum disorders needs assessment report. Public Health Institute of Scotland: Glasgow.

Richardson M 2000 How we live: participatory research with six people with learning disabilities. Journal of Advanced Nursing 32(6):1383-1395.

Scottish Executive 2000 The same as you? A review of services for people with learning disabilities. Edinburgh: The Stationery Office.

Scottish Executive 2002 Promoting Health, Supporting Inclusion: The national review of the contribution of all nurses and midwives to the care and support of people with learning disabilities. Edinburgh: The Stationery Office.

Scottish Executive 2003 Home at Last? The Report on Hospital Closure Service Reprovision Sub Group – The Same As You? Edinburgh: The Stationery Office.

Scottish Executive 2006a Having your say? The follow up report to The same as you? review of services for people with learning disabilities – report on advocacy. Edinburgh: The Stationery Office.

Scottish Executive 2006b Follow up report of The same as you? review of services for people with learning disabilities – report on children's services. Edinburgh: The Stationery Office.

Scottish Executive 2006c A follow up report of the same as you? review of services for people with learning disabilities – report on day services. Edinburgh: The Stationery Office.

Scottish Executive 2006d Autistic Spectrum Disorders Needs Assessment Report: Scottish Executive Report on Implementation and Next Steps. Edinburgh: The Stationery Office.

Scottish Executive 2006 Changing Lives: Report of the 21st Century Review of Social Work. Edinburgh: The Stationery Office.

Scottish Executive 2007 Evaluation of the Implementation of Local Area Co-ordination in Scotland. Edinburgh: The Stationery Office.

Scottish Intercollegiate Guidelines Network 2007 Assessment, diagnosis and clinical interventions for children and young people with autism spectrum disorders. Edinburgh: SIGN.

Social Work Inspection Agency 2007 Multi-agency Inspection of Service for People with Learning Disabilities in Ayrshire. Edinburgh: SWIA.

Walmsley J 2001 Normalisation, emancipatory research and inclusive research in learning disability. Disability and Society 16(2):187-205.

Walmsley J 2004a Involving users with learning difficulties in health improvement: lessons for inclusive learning disability research. Nursing Inquiry 11(1):54-64.

Walmsley J 2004b Inclusive learning disability research: the (nondisabled) researcher's role. British Journal of Learning Disabilities 32:65-71.

Welsh Assembly 2002 Fulfilling the promises: proposals for a framework for services for people with learning disabilities.Welsh Assembly, Cardiff.

Whitaker S, Read S 2006 The prevalence of psychiatric disorders among people with intellectual disabilities: An analysis of the literature. Journal of Applied Research in Intellectual Disabilities 19:330-345.

Will 'Equal Lives' be achieved in Northern Ireland?

Owen Barr and Members of the Users Council, Compass Advocacy Group

5

INTRODUCTION

Since the turn of this century all four countries in the United Kingdom have produced major reviews of policy in relation to services for people with intellectual disabilities. First, Scotland (Same as You?; Scottish Executive 2000), then England (Valuing People; Department of Health 2001), followed by Wales (Fulfilling the Promises; 2002) and then Northern Ireland (Equal Lives; 2005). The titles given to these documents have highlighted the importance of recognising the citizenship of people with intellectual disabilities. All four policy reviews provide clear recommendations for action and clearly set challenges for individuals and organisations in future service delivery to respond to.

As the chapters within this section have demonstrated progress in realising the vision of future services has been mixed and often not as quick as originally thought. This chapter commences with an overview of the changing structure of health and social services in Northern Ireland. It then outlines the involvement of people with intellectual disabilities in the process of policy review in Northern Ireland which led to the publication of Equal Lives (Department of Health, Social Services and Public Safety 2005). Following that the chapter then moves on to give an account of the feedback of a conference organised by Compass Advocacy Network to discuss the Equal Lives report (www.compasspeople.org). This conference provided over 100 people with intellectual disabilities opportunities to hear about the Equal Lives policy review and to highlight the practical developments they felt were needed for the vision provided within 'Equal Lives' to become the reality in future services.

NORTHERN IRELAND: AN OVERVIEW

Northern Ireland is one of the four countries which make up the United Kingdom and shares a land border with the Republic of Ireland. The 2001 population census reported that 1.7 million people were living in Northern Ireland, of which 16 366 have been reported as having an intellectual disability (McConkey et al 2003).

The overall prevalence rate of people with intellectual disabilities in Northern Ireland was 9.71 per 1000 people, although prevalence rates varied across different age groups and reflected the pattern within most developed

LIVERPOOL JOHN MOORES UNIVERSITY
AVRIL ROBARTS LRC
TEL: 0151 231 3179

countries which showed higher numbers of young people with intellectual disabilities in comparison to older people. The reported prevalence rates across age groups varied from 16.3 for people 19 years old or less, to 10.2 for people aged 20–34 years, and 7.0 for people aged 35–49 years, to 4.5 for those people aged 50 years or older (McConkey et al 2003).

As noted in other policy reviews within the United Kingdom the numbers of people with intellectual disabilities are expected to increase by 1% a year over the next 10–15 years. Not only will this lead to a higher number of people with intellectual disabilities, it is also expected to lead to a higher proportion of people with complex health needs, both younger people requiring support for their complex physical healthcare needs who will increasingly live into adulthood and older people who were previously healthy but develop complex health needs as they grow older (Department of Health, Social Services and Public Safety 2005). While accepting services for people with intellectual disabilities should not be underpinned solely by attention to the physical or mental healthcare needs, it is important to recognise the degree to which the complexity of healthcare needs are changing and the implications of this will require future intellectual disability services and wider mainstream health, social services, education and housing services to be able to respond effectively to this challenge.

Within Northern Ireland, health and social services have been provided within a combined structure of heath and social services boards and health and services trusts, as distinct from arrangements elsewhere in the United Kingdom in which health services are provided by Health Trusts and social services are the responsibility of Local Authorities.

NORTHERN IRELAND: A TIME OF CHANGE

At the time of writing this chapter in August 2008, Northern Ireland is very much in a state of flux, as three major changes are underway; these are the reinstatement of the Northern Assembly, the Review of Public Administration and the implementation of the Bamford Review of Mental Health and Learning Disability.

The first Northern Ireland Legislative Assembly met in 1999, following elections in 1998. However, this initial Assembly had largely a 'start–stop' period during which negotiations and disagreements continued. Due to a series of factors this Assembly was suspended in October 2002. Following a further election in 2003, there was a review of the Belfast Agreement, and a period of further negotiations between political parties. Following another election the Northern Ireland Assembly was reinstated on the 7th May 2007 (http://www.niassembly.gov.uk). The effect of this has been the appointment of locally elected politicians as Members of the Legislative Assemble (MLAs), some of whom took up ministerial positions, including a Minister of Health. A key area which the Assembly will have to make decisions about will be the implementation of the Bamford Review, including the Equal Lives report which specifically outlines the vision of future services for people with intellectual disabilities and their families.

In June 2002, the Northern Ireland Assembly (prior to suspension) instigated a review of all structures and systems involved in public administration within Northern Ireland. This included a review of the work of over 150 public bodies covering areas such as health and social services, education, local councils and education, and housing. The outcome of this review was the largest restructuring of public bodies within the history of Northern Ireland, including the role of The Department of Health, Social Services and Public Safety, the Health and Social Services Boards as well as the Health and Social Services Trusts. This review has resulted in the setting up of one Health and Social Care Authority (planned from April 2008), the removal of four Health and Social Services Boards (previously in commissioning roles) and the merging of 18 previous Health and Social Services Trusts into five larger Trusts (from April 2007). While the five new Health and Social Services Trusts came into being on 1st April 2007, at the time of writing this chapter (August 2008) the plans to remove the four Health and Social Services Boards is being further considered by the Minister for Health, Social Services Public Safety in the Northern Legislative Assembly. It is now unlikely that the necessary arrangements will be in place to remove these Boards in April 2008 as previously timetabled. In addition, seven Local Commissioning Groups are being set up and these will work with the new Health and Social Care Authority to commission health and social services across Northern Ireland; their development will be to some degree linked to the changes in the Boards as these are the current commissioning structures.

The Bamford Review of Mental Health and Learning Disability (N. Ireland)

Northern Ireland, although part of the United Kingdom, has specific regional legislation and policy documents relating to services for people with intellectual disabilities, and is not governed by the many legislation and policy documents in place within Scotland, England or Wales. In 1995 a review of policy for people with a learning disability was undertaken in Northern Ireland and this was the first policy document in the United Kingdom to specifically identify inclusion as a major policy objective, stating that 'the aim of Government policy for people with a learning disability should be inclusion. It is for Government and society to include people with a learning disability as they would any other member of society and to accept them for who they are and the way they are' (Department of Health and Social Services 1995:44).

In 2002, learning disability policy and legislation underwent a further major review as an integral part of the Bamford Review of Mental Health and Learning Disability in Northern Ireland. The terms of reference for the Bamford Review are listed in Box 5.1. As the title of the Bamford Review suggests it had a remit to consider mental health and learning disability services, as distinct from being a specific learning disability review such as those undertaken in Scotland, England and Wales. The work of the Bamford Review was undertaken by 10 Expert Committees, one of which focused on services for people with learning disability. In September 2005, this committee published a specific policy document on services for people with learning disabilities and their families entitled 'Equal Lives'. The objectives and recommendations within this report apply to all services being provided to

Box 5.1   Terms of reference for the Bamford Review

1. To carry out an independent review of the effectiveness of current policy and service provision relating to mental health and learning disability, and of the Mental Health (Northern Ireland) Order 1986.
2. To take into account:
   - the need to recognise, preserve, promote and enhance the personal dignity of people with mental health needs or a learning disability and their carers;
   - the need to promote positive mental health in society;
   - relevant legislative and other requirements, particularly relating to human rights, discrimination and equality of opportunity;
   - evidence-based best practice developments in assessment, treatment and care regionally, nationally and internationally;
   - the need for collaborative working among all relevant stakeholders both within and outside the health and personal social services sector;
   - the need for comprehensive assessment, treatment and care for people with a mental health need or a learning disability who have offended or are at risk of offending; and
   - issues relating to incapacity.
3. To make recommendations regarding future policy, strategy, service priorities and legislation, to reflect the needs of users and carers. (www.rmhldni.gov.uk)

people with learning disabilities and their families, not just those provided by learning disability services (Department of Health, Social Services and Public Safety 2005).

However, the combining of a review on mental health and learning disabilities was acknowledged has having two key disadvantages by the Learning Disability Committee undertaking the review and was not their preferred option. These concerns centred on, firstly, the potential for confusion between people with mental health problems and people with learning disabilities. Secondly, that key aspects of the lives of people with learning disabilities were potentially being addressed by one of the other nine committees meeting within the Review which were not specific to learning disabilities. This risked that some key learning disability issues may not be fully addressed and issues relevant to people with learning disabilities being fragmented across a number of individual committee reports (Department of Health, Social Services and Public Safety 2005).

In response to these concerns the Equal Lives Committee within the wider Bamford Review sought to ensure regular contact between members of different committees and highlighted that all committees across the review must consider people with learning disabilities within their discussions. With hindsight the combination of the review of services for people with learning disabilities and people with mental health problems may have also brought some advantages, in so far as the need for all the Expert Committees to consider the needs of people with learning disabilities, their needs were clearly considered within a wide range of mental health committees which may not have occurred if a separate mental health review had been undertaken.

The involvement of people with learning disabilities: 'The Equal Lives Group'

A guiding principle which was identified as underpinning the Bamford Review was that there should be involvement and open access of users, volunteers, professionals, organisations, carers and other groups throughout the review process. A key goal of the Review Team was 'to ensure that user and carer partnership is intrinsic to the Review at all stages' (www.rmhldni.gov. uk). In order to facilitate the involvement of people with intellectual disabilities within the Learning Disability Expert Committee, a user reference group known as the 'Equal Lives Group' was set up. This consisted of 12 people with learning disabilities from different parts of Northern Ireland and three people to support them. The Equal Lives Group were asked by the Committee to gather information in the following areas:

- What supports do parents and children with a learning disability need?
- What types of housing and support are needed for people with a learning disability?
- How can we make sure that people with a learning disability get the best things to do in the daytime?
- What do older people with a learning disability need?
- How do we make sure that people with a learning disability get good help if they are sick?

The members of the group met five times to get to know each other and plan how they could contribute to the Review. As well as contributing their own views the Equal Lives Group held four consultations across Northern Ireland in order to gather the views of other people with intellectual disabilities. They also attended meetings of advocacy groups who had asked to speak with them, speaking with 130 people in all. The members of the Equal Lives Group held monthly meetings and had regular meetings with the Equal Lives Committee members in order to provide them with information from their consultations and discuss the progress of the Review. All documents produced by the Equal Lives Committee were also discussed with the members of the Equal Lives Group before being finalised. The Equal Lives Group also produced their own report entitled 'We Have a Dream' which captured the key points they wished to make in response to the questions they were asked to address by the Committee (www.rmhldni.gov.uk). Within this report the key points for action that were made are outlined below:

- Everybody should have a choice where they live and if they want to stay in their local area then they should be supported to.
- If people want to live on their own or with friends they should get the help they need to do that.
- All staff who work with people with a learning disability should get special training so that they understand how to respect people and know what to do to support people with a learning disability.

- Any time people are making decisions about services or support they should have to listen to people with a learning disability.
- We hope that the Review will make sure that there are more advocacy groups and more chances for people to speak out and be listened to. We do not think this happens enough and that is why things go wrong.
- 'People with disabilities should have the same opportunities as people without a disability'
  (Department of Health, Social Services and Public Safety 2004:24–25).

This group continues to be consulted in the development of strategies and action plans to implement the findings of the Bamford Review.

Equal Lives: the way forward

A draft of the Equal Lives Report was issued for consultation in late 2004. Following a period of consultation and some revisions the final report was issued in September 2005. The Report set out a vision of services to be achieved over a 15-year period, to achieve what has been referred to as a 20:20 vision of services which was underpinned by five core service values:

Citizenship: People with a learning disability are individuals first and foremost and each has a right to be treated as an equal citizen.

Social inclusion: People with a learning disability are valued citizens and must be enabled to use mainstream services and be fully included in the life of the community.

Empowerment: People with a learning disability must be enabled to actively participate in decisions affecting their lives.

Working together: Conditions must be created where people with a intellectual disability, families and organisations work well together in order to meet the needs and aspirations of people with a learning disability.

Individual support: People with a learning disability will be supported in ways that take account of their individual needs and help them to be as independent as possible. (Department of Health, Social Services and Public Safety 2005:6-7)

Twelve key objectives (see Box 5.2) and 74 recommendations for practical changes in services were identified as necessary for the vision of future services is to be realised.

PROGRESS TOWARDS THE VISION OF FUTURE SERVICES

Current services in Northern Ireland have continued to make progress as they were prior to the launch of Equal Lives; however, the progress on achieving the vision as outlined in Equal Lives is limited (Taggart 2007), largely influenced by three key aspects. Firstly, at the time of writing this chapter (August 2008) it has been 3 years since the Equal Lives report was launched, but yet it still not has been officially accepted as the government policy for service within Northern Ireland. This is a consequence in part to the suspension of

Box 5.2 Twelve key objectives within Equal Lives Report (DHSSPS 2005)

Children, young people and families

To ensure that families are supported to enjoy seeing their children develop in an environment that recognises and values their uniqueness as well as their contributions to society.

To ensure that children and young people with a learning disability get the best possible start in life and access opportunities that are available to others of their age.

Fuller lives

To ensure that the move into adulthood for young people with a learning disability supports their access to equal opportunities for continuing education, employment and training and that they and their families receive continuity of support during the transition period.

To enable people with a learning disability to lead full and meaningful lives in their neighbourhoods, have access to a wide range of social work and leisure opportunities and form and maintain friendships and relationships.

Accommodation

To ensure that all men and women with a learning disability have their home in the community, the choice of whom they live with and that, where they live with their family, their carers receive the support they need.

To ensure that an extended range of housing options is developed for men and women with a learning disability.

Health and wellbeing

To secure improvements in the mental and physical health of people with a learning disability through developing access to high quality health services that are as locally based as possible and responsive to the particular needs of people with a learning disability.

Growing older

To ensure that men and women with a learning disability are supported to age well in their neighbourhoods.

Ensuring personal outcomes

To enable people with a learning disability to have as much control as possible over their lives through developing person centred approaches in all services and ensuring wider access to advocacy and Direct Payments.

Enabling change

To ensure that health and social services staff are confident and competent in working with people with a learning disability.

Continued

Box 5.2   Twelve key objectives within Equal Lives Report (DHSSPS 2005)—cont'd

To ensure that staff in other settings develop their understanding and awareness of learning disability issues and the implications for their services.

Managing change
To promote improved joint working across sectors and settings in order to ensure that the quality of lives of people with a learning disability is improved and that the Equal Lives values and objectives are achieved.

the Northern Ireland Assembly, until May 2007. Secondly, although the previous Direct Rule Minister with responsibilities for health in place during 2005–2007 highlighted the need for action to be taken to support people with intellectual disabilities and their families he stopped short of officially accepting the Equal Lives Report. Thirdly, while the restructuring of services which is presently underway as a results of the implementation of the Review of Public Administration provides opportunities to take major steps forward by increasing the level of consistency across a smaller number of Trusts and Northern Ireland as a whole, it is difficult to develop and sustain momentum for change within such a state of flux. A consequence of the above set of circumstances is that action to develop services risks becoming reactive, in response to negative publicity in the media, rather than being focused on proactively delivering the vision outlined with Equal Lives (http://news.bbc. co.uk/1/hi/northern_ireland/6273627.stm).

On a more positive note, developments do continue to take place, and expectations of further positive developments have been raised with the new structures for health and social care becoming stabilised and starting to perform effectively. Opportunities for more locally focused decision making by locally accountable politicians are expected to increase through the reinstatement of the Northern Ireland Assembly to make decisions that will directly impact on services. Key decisions on funding affecting the implementation of Equal Lives were made in 2008 and that this will commence an era of further growth and sustained development.

At a strategic level three steps have been taken, although at the time of the conference only the first step had been taken, this was the appointment by the Minister for Health, Social Services and Public Safety in Northern Ireland of a Mental Health and Learning Disability Board in June 2007. This Board has been given the remit 'to advise and challenge him and will be one of the driving forces in delivering the Bamford reforms' (http://www.northernireland. gov.uk/news/news-dhssps/news-dhssps-280607-mcgimpsey-announces-appointments.htm accessed 1st July 2007).

In anticipation of a period of further development of services, Compass Advocacy Network, a regional advocacy group within Northern Ireland, felt it was important to provide an opportunity for people with intellectual disabilities to identify the practical changes they felt are necessary to improve their life experiences. In order to facilitate this, a conference entitled 'Stand

Up, Speak Up' was organised by the User Council of Compass Advocacy Network in June 2007 (www.compasspeople.org).

Since June 2007, three further steps have taken place, these were the announcement of the terms of reference for a Service Framework focusing on people with intellectual disabilities in October 2007. When this is completed it will be the only Service Framework specifically focused on people with intellectual disabilities in the United Kingdom (Box 5.3). The timeframe for this work is that a Learning Disability Service Framework consultation document will be received by the Department of Health, Social Services and Public Safety by the 30th June 2008. Then, in January 2008, the Ministers in the Northern Ireland Assembly agreed a Programme for Government and

---

Box 5.3   Aim and scope of the Learning Disability Service Framework

Aim
The overall aim of the Learning Disability Service Framework is to improve the health and wellbeing of people with a learning disability and their families in Northern Ireland through promoting social inclusion, reduce inequalities in health and wellbeing, and improve HSC quality of care.

Of particular importance is the need to value the uniqueness of the individual and to promote integration into society so that individuals with learning disabilities can participate in the families and communities in which they live and can access the full range of opportunities open to everyone else.

Achievement of these aims goes beyond traditional health and social care boundaries and is strongly influenced by population/individual attitudes and behaviours, and the contribution of carers and other sectors.

Scope
The Learning Disability Service Framework will promote partnership working and the need for multidisciplinary assessment, diagnosis, treatment, ongoing care and regular review. It will promote the independence of the individual and will recognise the need to support the family/carer throughout the life of the individual, where appropriate, especially during the period of transition from childhood to adolescence and from adolescence to adulthood. It will focus on supporting equity of access to primary, secondary and specialist services appropriate to the needs of the individual and the family, in order to promote and maintain healthy living and prevent disease. The Learning Disability Service Framework will include specific standards for:

Children
- challenging behaviour.
- complex physical health care and social care needs.

Continued

Box 5.3 Aim and scope of the Learning Disability Service Framework—cont'd

- transitional arrangements from:
  - hospital to home;
  - home to preschool and school;
  - childhood to adolescence; and
  - adolescence to adulthood.
- supporting children and families:
  - enhancing the interface between social care provision and educational needs;
  - social and leisure activities;
  - lifestyle choices including diet and physical activity; and
  - respite care.

Adolescence
- enhancing physiological and psychological wellbeing.
- developing and maintaining positive mental health.
- promoting social care provision which maximises opportunities for vocational training.
- promoting independence in decision-making in preparation for transition from adolescence to adulthood.

Adulthood
- supporting individuals:
  - enabling choice and independence.
  - promoting social, educational, employment and leisure activities; and
  - multi-agency engagement on accommodation and housing needs.
- complex health and social care needs:
  - prevention, early intervention and management of comorbidities, e.g. coronary heart disease, respiratory disease and mental health conditions; and
- supporting people as they grow older
- supporting families:
  - respite care
  - support for carers in their changing roles; and
  - coping with bereavement.

corresponding funding. The Minster for Health, Social Services and Public Safety has highlighted the importance of services for people with intellectual disabilities within this Programme for Government, stating:

'Mental health and learning disability services have been my first priority. The funding I have received will allow me to make real progress with the Bamford recommendations. As well as doubling the numbers of long stay mental health and learning disability patients to be resettled in the community, there will be a considerable increase in the numbers of community-based staff and in the number of respite places. This will make a real and lasting difference to patients,

carers and families in an area which has too long been neglected and underfunded.'
http://www.northernireland.gov.uk/news/news-dhssps/news-dhssps-220108-extra-funding-for.htm

In July 2008 the DHSSPS response to the Bamford Review was issued for consultation (www.dhsspsnl.gov.uk).

However, as of August 2008, there still has been no official acceptance or response to the Equal Lives Report.

Organisation of the conference

The conference was organised and managed by the Compass Advocacy Network's User Council of 12 adults with intellectual disabilities, supported by members of the network. The purpose of the conference was to provide people with intellectual disabilities attending the conference the opportunity to give their views on the changes in their experience that would be necessary for the recommendations to become a reality in their lives. Invitations to the conference were sent out through the Advocacy Network's contacts and over 100 people with intellectual disabilities attended the conference.

The User Council selected a number of areas from the Equal Lives recommendations to hold workshops on. These included health, transport, housing, and employment & training. These areas were selected as the members of the User Council felt these would be most pertinent to their lives and those of the people attending the event. Each workshop followed the same format and commenced with members of the User Council introducing the topic and explaining the process to be followed, assisted where they felt necessary by a facilitator. After that people attending the workshop were asked to answer the following questions in relation to the title of their workshop:

1. What do you think this is (means)?
2. Why do you think it is important to you?
3. Do you have access to this?
4. Do you think this area can work for people with intellectual disabilities?
5. Do you think access to this area is the same for a person with intellectual disability as a person who does not have intellectual disability?
6. Is there any way you think this area could be improved to help you?

Feedback from workshops

The feedback from the workshops is presented below using each of the six key questions as a framework and drawing on the discussions across the four workshops topics.

What do you think this is (means)?

Overall, the people participating in the focus groups were able to explain in their own words what the titles of the workshops meant and give practical examples in relation to housing, transport, training and employment. Housing was considered 'the place where I live'… 'the place where I have a room' and the 'home is where I live at the minute'. A wide range of examples for transport were given, including 'train, car, scooter, motorbike, bicycle, boat, also walking, jogging and running were included. Transport was summarised as 'travel from one place to another'. Employment training was also seen as concrete activities including 'getting a job', and 'learn new skills… prepare for work'.

The majority of participants in the healthcare workshops explained healthcare as 'looking after your self', 'to make people well'… 'feel better' and 'to make sure you feel alright'. However, the term 'healthcare' caused some uncertainty for a number of participants, who were 'not sure what the term means', and were unclear exactly what was involved. Once the term healthcare was clarified in relation to the people involved in providing these services participants were clearer about what was included. Participants then added to this list and demonstrated their knowledge of a wide range of health professionals such as, GP, nurse, dentist, optician, chiropodist, psychologists and behaviour therapists. In addition they also included, 'fire people, hairdresser, well women clinics, cancer nurses, occupational therapists, social workers and blind guide dog', which appeared to indicate some lack of clarity around the traditionally perceived boundaries of healthcare, even within a joint health and social care structure as in Northern Ireland and some participants still considered the term 'healthcare' to be jargon.

Why do you think it is important to you?

After establishing what the name of the workshop covered, participants provided a wide range of reasons under each heading as to why each area was important, for example transport 'gets you to work' and 'you can get out and do things', and housing was important as it was necessary to 'know you had a roof over your head'. Participants highlighted that employment and training were important as these provided the opportunities 'to learn life skills… meet new people… make new friends', which was important as some participants talked about how they 'get bored at home'. They discussed how having opportunities for training and employment were important as these made people 'happy when they are good at something' and provided opportunities 'to make money'.

Feedback from participants also demonstrated how these areas are interdependent and identified overarching reasons for their importance, with housing, health and transport all being considered necessary to 'keep you safe' and 'help you feel better about yourself'… and 'be happy… keep you right'. Perhaps healthcare was considered most important in this aspect as it was necessary 'so you don't die… live longer'.

Do you have access to this?

Across the different workshops people reported access to all areas of services as they had interpreted them. The majority of participants lived with family members, with only one living in residential accommodation and one in supported accommodation. In respect of transport all participants in the workshop had access to cars, trains, buses, and all but one reported travelling on an aeroplane and two had not travelled on a boat. When discussing training and employment participants felt that in particular there were 'not enough opportunities especially for people living in the country', that 'transport is a big problem', concluding that there was 'still a lot to be done'.

Do you think this area can work for people with intellectual disabilities?

Across the workshops, participants appeared to feel strongly that the topics discussed within the workshops were important to them and that these areas should also work effectively for people with intellectual disabilities. People gave examples of where services were working, such as 'getting their medicine from the chemist', and as well as restating many of the examples provided earlier when discussing access to services. Several participants were clear in their views that they had the 'same needs as everybody else' and asked 'Why not? What is different about us?' and 'no reason why we 'can't' do it'.

Do you think access to this area is the same for a person with intellectual disability as a person who does not have intellectual disability?

When discussing the extent of access for people with intellectual disabilities it became clear that participants believed they had the same right to access services as people who do not have intellectual disabilities, but across all the workshops many participants had experienced difficulties in relation to achieving access to services. People found they often needed the assistance of other people such as a family member or staff member to access services such as transport and healthcare. These people organised appointments and provided the support necessary to use public transport by checking timetables and prompting people on which service to use.

Access to healthcare was identified as problematic at times with participants across two workshops stating that 'Dr is often too busy and you have to wait to be seen', 'it is hard to get an appointment' and 'transport can be a problem'. Given the stated difficulties, people accessing healthcare reported they were often accompanied by a family or staff member, which participants in the focus groups valued, as one participant explained, 'my sister gets my appointments' and 'sometimes other people can come to appointments and this helps me' but quickly qualified this by saying 'the person has a choice about who comes into the room to see the GP'. When discussing training and employment, participants reported that 'people don't understand our needs', and 'from experience when people have 'problems' employers don't understand our needs'.

Is there any way you think this area could be improved to help you?

Participants were asked to talk about their thoughts or suggestions on how services could be improved. The focus was on the wider services of transport, health, housing, training & employment rather than only intellectual disability services. During the earlier discussions within the workshops, participants had highlighted areas of difficulties in accessing services and their suggestions largely addressed how these may be overcome.

Participants appeared to recognise that they may present extra challenges to services as noted in comments such as, 'it is harder for a person with learning disabilities, than someone else with no learning disability', 'harder to make myself understood' and 'it can be difficult for us to understand'. However, participants also recognised that services at times did not make the necessary adjustments and commented that 'it can be difficult to understand everything they are talking about especially if they (healthcare staff) are in a hurry'. Perhaps the key area for change was twofold and captured by the participant who stated that 'we need people to speak up and people need to listen'.

The suggestions for improvement often related to participants' previous experiences and were very practical in nature and perhaps may not have been as obvious to people without intellectual disabilities who will have different experiences in accessing and using services. Participants felt their suggestions could provide potential solutions to difficulties in accessing services (Box 5.4).

The above suggestions appear realistic and could provide a starting place for services who are seeking to translate broader policy aims and objectives into practical changes in how their services are promoted, organised and

---

Box 5.4   Participants' suggestions for areas for change in services

Transport
Timetables needed in larger print.
Need to explain the 24-hour clock, better if 12-hour clock used.
Time keeping is important, sometimes these are late.

Health
More time required.
Need to know more about mainstream services, such as dentists, psychologists, counselling services.
Need more information packs, clear information about Accident and Emergency and surgical wards.
Staff need more training and more contact with people who have learning disabilities.

Housing
Need to know more about options available to people.
'People should have more choice and be able to spend their own money and make their own decisions.'

Training & employment
Need more support in our jobs.
Need more opportunities.
Need help with transport getting to and from work.
People could come into school and tell us what is happening out there.
More support in our jobs and looking for jobs.
Receiving money in our jobs can cause barriers.

---

delivered. The clear ability of people with intellectual disabilities to identify practical issues as they had experienced them and be able when given the opportunities and support to make suggestions is also an important lesson arising from the workshops.

CONCLUSION

In returning to the question set at the start of this chapter about whether the aspirations of the Equal Lives document have been achieved in Northern Ireland, the answer is that the document remains a vision and sets the direction for future service developments. However, at the time of writing this chapter little real progress had occurred in the development of new services, in part due to the hiatus in a Legislative Assembly within Northern Ireland. With the Assembly now restored, high expectations exist that progress will occur and the first signs of this have been seen with the appointment of the Mental Health and Learning Disability Board in Northern Ireland.

However, further challenges remain to be effectively addressed. Key among these is a clear commitment from Assembly members and Ministers to accept and fund the vision presented within the Equal Lives; 2 years after publication of the policy no commitment has been made, although it is eagerly awaited.

Secondly to be effective, progress will have to occur in a wide range of services, including those discussed within the workshops, the necessary changes go well beyond changes that intellectual disability services can make. Therefore it will be essential that effective collaborative alliances are developed and should include people with intellectual disabilities, their families and carers, together with intellectual disability and so called 'mainstream' services in the statutory and independent sectors.

Finally, these collaborative alliances must lead to action and be more than talking shops. To make a difference in the lives of people with intellectual disabilities and their families, policy aims and objectives need to lead to practical changes. People with intellectual disabilities have clear ideas about types of changes needed; consistent messages about format of information and attitudes of people they are in contact with were also noted by the Equal Lives Group (Department of Health, Social Services and Public Safety 2004) during the Bamford Review and were echoed in the feedback from the participants in the workshops discussions.

People with intellectual disabilities are important allies in bringing about change. They often have clear ideas about practical changes, and also may have access to sources of power that are unlikely to be available to many staff in services. These include access to elected representatives and government ministers both as individual citizens and collectively. Through this they may be able to exert influence and pressure if needed in avenues, without the constraints that staff may feel, or are placed upon them in criticising services in which they work.

The policy review has been completed, the report written, and in many ways we are at the 'end of the beginning' in the process; what is needed now is action. The next few years will tell if the commitment and expectations of people with intellectual disabilities, their families and carers is going to be matched by the necessary funding and organisational changes that deliver

5

the integrated practical changes. These changes are needed across intellectual disability and wider services and must lead to real changes in the lives of people with intellectual disabilities which result in their expectations being met and delivering services that 'keep you safe'... 'get you from one place to another'... 'not being bored'... 'help you feel better about yourself' and 'make you happy when we are good at something'.

ACKNOWLEDGEMENT

I would like to thank the Members of the User Council, Compass Advocacy Network, Ballymoney, Northern Ireland for their contributions to this chapter:

Marion Kane	Evonne Leitch
Ursula Campbell	Hayley Allen
Robert Adams	Gerard McKendry
Conrad McFeely	Madeleine McKendry
Peter Maxwell	Darren Stewart
Adam Martin	Mark Gray
Alistair Kane	Alison McAleese
Iris McFetridge	http://www.compasspeople.org/

REFERENCES

Department of Health 2001 Valuing People. A new strategy for learning disability for 21st century. The Stationery Office, London.

Department of Health and Social Services 1995 Review of policy for people with a learning disability. Department of Health and Social Services, Belfast.

Department of Health, Social Services and Public Safety 2004 We have a dream. Messages from people with learning disabilities to the Review. Department of Health, Social Services and Public Safety, Belfast.

Department of Health, Social Services and Public Safety 2005 Equal Lives: Draft report of Learning Disability Committee. Department of Health, Social Services and Public Safety, Belfast.

McConkey R, Spollen M, Jamison J 2003 Administrative Prevalence of Learning Disability in Northern Ireland. A Report to the Department of Health, Social Services and Public Safety. DHSSPS, Belfast.

Scottish Executive 2000 The same as you? A review of the services for people with learning disabilities. Scottish Executive, Edinburgh.

Taggart L 2007 Service provision for people with learning disabilities and psychiatric disorders in Northern Ireland. Advances in Mental Health and Learning Disabilities 1(1): 17-20.

INTELLECTUAL DISABILITY AND SOCIAL INCLUSION

Intellectual disabilities with mental health problems

Dave Ferguson

INTRODUCTION

It is readily acknowledged that people with intellectual disabilities do experience a similar range of mental health problems as those in the general population (Hardy & Bouras 2002, Raghavan 1996, Taggart & Slevin 2006). People with intellectual disabilities are more at risk of mental ill-health than the general population and require innovative approaches from support services regarding assessment and treatment.

The notion of where and how people receive treatment or the specific service response in meeting` their individual needs has been the topic for discussion for some time. The emphasis generally being on specialist intellectual disability provision, use of mainstream services or a mix of both.

Valuing People (2001) emphasises that mainstream services should be accessible for people who have a learning disability in the same way as the rest of the population. In particular, it makes specific reference to the mental health needs of people with a learning disability:

> 'The National Service Framework for Mental Health applies to all adults of working age. A person who has a learning disability and a mental illness should therefore expect to be able to access services and be treated in the same way as anyone else.'
>
> Department of Health 2001

It is suggested, however, that this group of individuals are disadvantaged when it comes to accessing mainstream services particularly with regard to services that lack the competencies and resources to be effective when delivering services (Gregory 2003).

This chapter aims to describe the efforts, practice developments and service responses led by me and my (professional and user) colleagues to promote an inclusive approach to service delivery and development. In this sense inclusion will be discussed not only in terms of using mainstream services but also in terms of user participation in service development and developing person-centred approaches to enable services to provide a coherent response to mental health care (Clinical Interface Protocol; Ferguson 2005:8).

The user voice is represented in the form of narratives. These were gathered via two user groups, who were approached asking for members who may be interested in telling their stories of using mental health services for this chapter. I met with users who expressed interest either in a group or individually and provided the necessary information in a variety of mediums to enable them to make an informed decision whether to proceed or not.

Each user met me individually (two individuals chose for a supporter to be with them) and a semi-structured interview took place. The interviews were handwritten by myself. Drafts were typed up and sent to the users for approval/amendment.

I met each user again to confirm that they were happy with the information they had shared to be used in the chapter. Consent forms provided by the publishers were then adapted (in consultation with a Speech and Language Therapist) and signed by the users. Two users chose to use pseudonyms. The information users have provided is supported by evidence from recent studies.

SETTING THE SCENE – USING MAINSTREAM SERVICES

The experiences of people with intellectual disabilities who have used mainstream services are mixed. This is what James had to say about his experience of using mainstream mental health services:

> 'I went into the hospital, I didn't like it. My mum and dad and social worker decided that I should go in – I wasn't asked. I was told I was going in because I was talking to myself. I wasn't very well.
>
> There was one TV and I wasn't allowed to see my family because I was ill. I had rough blankets, I was cold, and I was trying to get out because I didn't like it.
>
> I felt better after I had some tablets but I didn't know what they were for. I was in for a few weeks but I didn't know exactly what was happening to me – it made me feel unwell. I was drowsy and didn't feel in control. I didn't realise what was happening to me. I felt really unwell and was too ill to remember going in there. I remember wondering where I was.
>
> I felt looked after but I don't want to go back there. I think the doctors and nurses were able to look after me because my community nurse helped to teach them about me. I was told I had depression. I spent a lot of time in bed.
>
> I think my family should have been allowed to see me. It might have made me feel better sooner.'

Clearly this is a unique experience, and for James a particularly negative one. He was not included in decisions affecting his care, he was not able to retain contact with his family and some of the environmental conditions were not to his liking.

Let us look at an extract from Karen's story:

> 'I thought I wasn't ill enough to have to go into hospital but people said I should go in. I didn't like it – it was horrible – it is not your home – all around there is illness and that made me feel worse. The staff were reasonable although some didn't have the patience with people with learning disabilities but some did. They have to deal with a lot of ill people.
>
> A Learning Disability Nurse came to see me once a week and this made things better. Eventually I did feel happier with the decision that was made; I felt more in control when I got better. I felt safe and knew I was going to get well again.'

All service users' experiences will be unique. Karen's experience was different to James' and individual to her but there are some similarities, namely the support the mainstream services received from the Community Learning Disability Nurse. In my experience when an intellectual disability practitioner facilitates the specialist knowledge often required to enable mainstream services to provide care for this client group, the user outcome is generally more positive. Promoting inclusion is often led by an intellectual disability practitioner; however the message to mental health colleagues is that neither mental health nor intellectual disability services can achieve this on their own. Both need to play an active role.

Both James and Karen felt disempowered and not having control at the time of their admission and this is not unique to people with intellectual disabilities (Scior & Lango 2005).

I would suggest that people with intellectual disabilities are often 'integrated' into mainstream services rather than included in its truest sense. Douds (2003) questions how quality integrated services can be delivered to people with mental health needs. He suggests that mainstream mental health services have often not responded to the needs of people with an intellectual disability, that there is often the consequence of poor planning, making it difficult for people to access.

The journey as well as the destination service users reach has to be an important consideration. Chaplin (2004) undertook a review to inquire if there were better outcomes for users in mainstream or in specialist services. He concluded that there was no particular evidence to favour the use of mainstream or specialist mental health services but specialist services provided a better user outcome than mainstream provision.

Chaplin also found that staff working in mainstream services perceive they lack training and experience in the mental health needs of people who have an intellectual disability and this is implied in a paper by Xenitidis et al (2004). They suggest a workforce with specialist skills and knowledge when working with this specific client group will make the patient experience a more positive one for all concerned.

There would still appear to be a lack of understanding of the mental health needs of people with intellectual disabilities, lack of specific training as well as communication difficulties between clinician and user (Chan et al 2004). This issue has been raised indirectly in James' and Karen's narratives.

Priest & Gibbs (2004) suggest people with intellectual disabilities will often receive poor care in mainstream mental health service provision. One reason is that they often require longer stays giving the impression that their needs may be more complex than other patients whose journey is swifter through the inpatient process.

Alexander et al (2002) demonstrated that psychiatrists in intellectual disabilities had concerns about the needs of people who had mental health needs and intellectual disability. They suggest those who used mainstream services would be marginalised in comparison with high profile demands of severe mental illness and personality disorder. This concern appeared to be further increased as there is no specific reference in the National Service Framework for Mental Health (Department of Health 1999) to those who have an intellectual disability.

Intellectual disabilities with mental health problems

Hall et al (2006) suggest that people who have intellectual disabilities are rarely a priority for mainstream mental health services and although Chaplin (2004) suggests that the advantages of general psychiatric services will include lack of discrimination and stigma, care may be below an optimum standard because mental health professionals could lack the necessary training, knowledge, skills and attitudes when working with people who have an intellectual disability.

There is however some literature that would suggest access to mainstream services can be successful (Chan et al 2004, Gibson 2007) and this requires a number of initiatives to be effective. The next sections in this chapter will explore how I and my colleagues have improved access to mainstream services.

DEVELOPING A CLINICAL INTERFACE PROTOCOL

In response to some of the inclusion challenges mentioned, I led an initiative aimed to improve the working relationships between the mainstream mental health and intellectual disability services and thereby improve the user experience though the development of a clinical interface protocol. This section will discuss its development and ongoing work.

A key aspect of Valuing People (2001) relates to the importance of close collaboration between adult mental health and intellectual disability services, with the provision of clear protocols outlining joint working. It also states that each local service should have access to an assessment and treatment resource for people with significant intellectual disability and mental health needs who cannot be appropriately admitted to general psychiatric wards, even where there is the provision of specialist intellectual disability support.

Unfortunately for some there are inconsistent approaches to patterns of provision – mental health services refusing to accept people because of their intellectual disability and intellectual disability services refusing to accept people because of their mental health (Coyle 2000).

Disputes between mainstream and specialist intellectual disability services have been reported and a challenge for users and their carers is that organisational boundaries do not hinder access to the essential expertise and support these services provide (Hollins & Courtenay 2000). Internationally, services for this client group would appear to have developed in many different ways. As previously mentioned Valuing People has proposed that all mainstream hospital services are available to people with intellectual disabilities (Chaplin 2004). It suggests that clear local protocols are in place for collaboration between Specialist Learning Disability Services and Specialist Mental Health Services.

The Clinical Interface Protocol (Ferguson 2004, 2005) was led by the author within Hampshire Partnership NHS Trust. It was developed with the intellectual disability and adult mental health directorates across two localities to apply to adults who have a diagnosed intellectual disability and who experience mental illness. It clarifies the operational arrangements between the two directorates to ensure service users are seen efficiently and are supported from both or either service as appropriate. It had particular poignancy for those users which neither service would accept or, in some cases, take responsibility for.

Both Valuing People, A New Strategy for Learning Disability for the 21st Century (2001) and National Service Framework for Mental Health Services (1999) have indicated how services should be developed for people who have an intellectual disability and mental health problems. They recommend services should be:

- Integrated as far as possible into local generic services
- Easy to access
- Have individualized assessments and care packages, including care plans under the Care Programme Approach
- Have an emphasis on prevention
- Have good working relationships with primary care services plus effective links with secondary and tertiary services
- Have partnership agreements between service users
- Promote service users and carer involvement
- Promote evidence based practice
- Provide assessment and intervention at home or in the least restrictive environment

A positive effect has been achieved through the support of influential clinicians and by clearly demonstrating the benefits of joint working and through action.

In a wider context, there is a challenge for the Local Implementation Teams (LITs) and the Partnership Boards to interpret and implement the centrally driven agenda which Valuing People *prescribes* but also *describes* the requirements for both intellectual disability and mental health services to offer better mental health care to service users. Therefore effective partnership working has to take place at the local level.

As implied through James' and Karen's narratives, there have been other challenges:

- Communication in its broadest sense can be a barrier for people who have an intellectual disability. Not just the communication inabilities of some service providers with users (e.g. not giving them information about their illness) but also the communication difficulties between service providers.
- Knowledge and skill base of some mental health clinicians would appear to focus on their qualifications rather than on their skills; however there are very positive approaches that are working – some that have been supported through additional training in intellectual disability approaches or by supporting and supervising mental health staff in the necessary skills required to work with this client group.

Only with a collaborative effort will services provide responsive mental health services to people who have both an intellectual disability and mental health problem. If services communicate well and share expertise appropriate responses will be enabled for this client group (Coyle 2000). Genuine partnership between organisations is key to improving services and this has to involve the user and carer – especially to ensure that service inclusion meets the needs of users in a person centred manner.

Partnership working will now be discussed in the next section of this chapter.

GREEN LIGHT TOOLKIT – INVOLVING AND INCLUDING USERS TOWARDS EFFECTIVE SERVICE CHANGE AT A LOCAL LEVEL

Green Light for Mental Health (2004) has been written in partnership between the National Institute for Mental Health in England (NIMHE) and the Valuing People Support Team (VPST). The toolkit claims that support for people with intellectual disabilities who have mental health problems is not the exclusive responsibility of just one service. People will receive support from local primary care, mental health, intellectual disability, public and voluntary sector services, and others. The toolkit determines what all of those services can do to improve mental health support for people with intellectual disabilities.

In recent years it has become more recognised that service users can offer useful and unique insights into the development and planning of services based upon their experiences. Working in partnership with people with intellectual disabilities allows inclusion of service users' and carers' experience, which is recognised as crucial to building better services (Ferguson 2004).

Inclusion is not just about accessing or being integrated into services. User involvement in every step of the client journey is crucial to the overall quality of care provision. The Southampton Users Working Group have been actively working to improve the experience for users, e.g. by advising on service development and producing information leaflets for other service users.

However, there is a salutary warning from a past inspection report (Social Services Inspectorate 1998) as communication and consultation arrangements were heavily criticised by service users and their carers when involved in consultations about improvements to services. Many complained about consultation fatigue and tokenism and reported seeing little effect of their involvement as services were more concerned with meeting statistical activity and performance targets rather than driving change from a user perspective.

A key recommendation from this criticism in the report was that organisations must demonstrate how the views of service users have affected the way in which services are delivered – as well as how ideas about new services include ideas from users and carers (Social Services Inspectorate 1998).

When interviewed for the Green Light Project, users in Southampton said that when they were unwell services would generally be mobilised; however, when they become well services tended to withdraw. This meant that as a result of service withdrawal, some users would present themselves (or via a referrer) to locality teams in quick succession (Patterson 2006 Report on the Southampton City green light toolkit service evaluation of mental health services for people with intellectual disabilities). This highlighted the need for services to be more person centred in their mental health care to people with intellectual disabilities and heightened the importance of the recovery agenda. The principles that are important here are those that are meaningful to service users. This would involve being positive about change and promoting social inclusion for mental health users and carers. These can be highlighted as:

- working in partnership with service users (and/or carers) to identify realistic life goals and enabling them to achieve them;
- stressing the value of social inclusion;

- emphasising the need for professionals to be optimistic about the possibility of positive individual change.

In response to this a workshop was organised to address better person-centred mental health care. Invited to the workshop were users and their carers, a carer's consultant, WRAP coordinator for Hampshire as well as health and adult service practitioners.

The workshop found there to be a number of recovery issues concerning how users could be more involved and in control of their care. This required address on an individual and wider service user perspective and took into account the following:

- Care Programme Approach
- Partnership
- Expertise of staff
- User experience – planning when well

From this a working group of users and service providers developed to explore how recovery should and could be incorporated into intellectual disability practice.

The recovery model used in Hampshire Partnership NHS Trust originates from the work of Copeland (2002) and Wellness Recovery Action Plan (WRAP). The model used is designed for users to take personal control of their recovery, using their own expertise and experience. By writing a WRAP they can help professionals to tell them how services can help them more effectively. It empowers users by enabling them to look more closely at their illness and to achieve a greater sense and achievement of how they can stay well.

Below, Sharon shares some insight into her own illness, the signs she recognises of her mental health deterioration and what she has learnt to stay as well as possible:

'Sometimes I am disturbed and need to be on my own. Sometimes felt people couldn't hear me and that my voice was funny. I was hiding in my bedroom. I feel all tense inside and then it feels like a butterfly in my stomach. It feels like it's the colour red and its ready to burst out. Sometimes it frightens me.

I am able to talk things through with the Community Team. I have had a CPA but I am now discharged but I have a review for my physical health in case it affects my mental health.

I have a say in my mental health treatment. I more or less sort myself out now – I take the tablets myself and know if I miss them I will not feel well.'

Sharon highlights here that illness can be time limited and that she has taken back control of her mental health. However no person is an island and recovery is not an outcome but a journey (Repper & Perkins 2003).

WRAP is currently being piloted with people who have an intellectual disability and mental health needs and gaining their views on layout, communication media and effectiveness in practice. As this model is being implemented across the adult mental health services in Hampshire it is another system, like

Intellectual disabilities with mental health problems

CPA, that clinicians in both mental health and intellectual disability services can use with this client group. The advantage of this will be that when users have developed their WRAP, whatever mental health service they may need to use within Hampshire will be familiar with the process and will lead to future service responses being more person centred. Such a partnership can be empowering for both user and provider.

Below, Patterson (2006:18) discusses how service users were included in the Green Light interview process:

'The Green Light Toolkit suggests someone with a learning disability would be ideally placed to carry out the interviews for the service user surveys, with appropriate training and support. This notion correlated with the Learning Disabilities Research and Development Strategy for Hampshire Partnership Trust (Ferguson 2005). Members of the service users' working group were asked if they would like to help carry out interviews for the project and two users were interested in contributing. Plans were made for users to be paid for their work and training was organized by the project worker and the Patient Advocacy & Liaison Service (PALS).

Training sessions were organized and were focused on talking about the questions that users thought were important to ask about people's experiences and what would be the best way to help the interviewers to ask questions. The questions were then typed up in large print with instructions for asking more elaborate questions typed in red. The interviewers felt this would be better because they could read the questions off the sheet in an interview. The interviewers thought of other questions that could be asked of people to find out about their experiences of mental health and learning disability.

Some role plays of interview situations were used to give the interviewers practice at asking questions and waiting for a response. The issues of consent and confidentiality were discussed and role plays were used to illustrate situations that might arise in the interviewing. For example, a participant who became upset answering questions and the interviewer asked if she would like to stop the interview.'

Whatever the directives may be from the Government, services need to be aware of the tensions and difficulties which could arise when listening to the views of service users and complying with governmental targets. However, one of the clear benefits in the Green Light Project was that user-interviewers were able to ask questions about participant's day to day lives in a more understanding way than the project worker because they were asking about topics they had personal experience of.

Achievements of the Green Light Toolkit in Southampton City

- Agreement of a local clinical interface protocol between Adult Mental Health and Learning Disabilities services
- Development of a protocol for referrals from Primary Care to Adult Mental Health and/or Learning Disabilities services
- Formal implementation of the Care Programme Approach to National Service Framework standards by Learning Disability services for people with mental health and intellectual disability needs

- Forming a ' virtual team' of professionals from mental health and intellectual disability services who will work together with people who have a mental problem and who have an intellectual disability

Southampton Service User Working Group

Nationally there are a number of intellectual disability service user groups who advise services, some via Partnership Boards, and give clear pictures of their experiences of living with an intellectual disability and of the services they receive. This is in response to enabling people with intellectual disabilities to 'have their voices heard and have wider opportunities' (Department of Health 2001).

Involving service users in service developments can serve different purposes. Kelson (2001), in Lugon & Secker-Walker's publication, suggests there are individual as well as organisational advantages for client inclusivity but overall as a useful means for securing quality services for clients. Kelson is mindful that developing effective client involvement requires commitment, time, effort, skills and resources – something which I believe has been achieved with the Southampton Service User Working Group.

The user group meets on a monthly basis and comprises users who have both an intellectual disability and have experienced or do experience mental ill health. The group is facilitated by two clinicians and members are paid for the work they undertake. Maim explains what the benefits are to her of being in the group:

> 'I like being in the group.
> I like to talk about helping other people with their mental health problems.
> I like talking in the group because it helps me to feel better.
> I like talking with everybody.
> I get paid for doing the work to help staff who work with people with learning disabilities to do a better job for other people.
> I have been to London to speak at a meeting about the group.
> Being part of the group helps other people too.
> I have been helping to write a book about keeping well.
> I have been helping the (Green Light Toolkit) project to write a book about CPA for other people who have a learning disability.'

They have been instrumental in advising and developing a person centred Care Programme Approach with particular reference to their own experiences. Issues they are delivering on include:

- CPA process to include only people that are known to the service user – use names/photos and introduce people beforehand and their role.
- Format of meetings. These must be person centred with a choice of friend/advocate to support if required.
- Developing a user-friendly CPA leaflet and advising into policy developments.
- Talking to and training staff groups across the agencies and nationally.

I believe the group demonstrate the possibilities available to service users and providers. They have enabled services to reflect and learn from their experiences and affect change as a result.

CONCLUSION

In this chapter I have discussed and described the efforts, practice developments and service responses to promote an inclusive approach to service delivery and development for people who have an intellectual disability and mental health problems.

The inclusion agenda underlines the importance of equality and empowerment. It is important to recognise that we all bring diverse yet valuable contributions to service delivery and development. Some individuals have shared their personal experiences of using services, emphasising that everyone's experience will be different whether it be positive or negative. Contributing to the development of person centred services is key to the inclusion agenda as this helps providers to understand how they should be more effective in service delivery and also enables users to develop their experiences to benefit others.

REFERENCES

Alexander R, Regan A, Gangadharan S, Bhaumik S 2002 Psychiatry of learning disability – a future with mental health? Psychiatric Bulletin 26:299-301.

Chan J, Hudson C, Vulic C 2004 Services for adults with intellectual disability and mental illness: are we getting it right? Australian e-Journal for the Advancement of Mental Health 3(1):1-6.

Chaplin R 2004 General psychiatric services for adults with intellectual disability and mental illness. Journal of Intellectual Disability Research 48(1):1-10.

Copeland M E 2002 Wellness recovery action plan. Peach Press, West Dummerston, USA.

Coyle D 2000 Meeting the needs of people with learning disabilities and mental health problems: a review. Mental Health Care 3(12):408.

Department of Health 1999 National service framework for mental health. HMSO, London.

Department of Health 2001 Valuing people: a new strategy for learning disability for the 21st century. HMSO, London.

Department of Health 2004 Green light for mental health: how good are your mental health services for people with learning disabilities? A service improvement toolkit. HMSO, London.

Douds F 2003 Integrated care for people with mental health and forensic needs. In: Brown M (ed) Learning disability: a handbook for integrated care. APS, p 234.

Ferguson D 2004 Learning disability research: a discussion paper. Learning Disability Practice 7(6):17-19.

Ferguson D 2005 Hampshire Partnership NHS Trust Learning Disability Research Strategy.

Gibson T 2007 Training opportunities in mental health and learning disabilities. Learning Disability Practice 10(1):35-36.

Gregory M 2003 Green light?: mental health services for people with a learning disability. Living Well 3(3):26.

Hall I, Higgins A, Parkes C et al 2006 The development of a new integrated mental health service for people with learning disabilities. British Journal of Learning Disabilities 34:82-83.

Hardy S, Bouras N 2002 The presentation and assessment of mental health in people with learning disabilities. Learning Disability Practice 5(3):33-38.

Hollins S, Courtenay K 2000 Issues and dilemmas for learning disability community psychiatric services. Mental Health Review 5(2):26-29.

Kelson M 2001 Patient involvement in clinical governance. In: Lugon M, Secker-Walker J (eds) Advancing clinical governance. The Royal Society of Medicine Press Ltd, pp 5-18.

National Institute for Mental Health for England 2005 NIMHE Guiding statement on recovery. DoH.

Patterson L 2006 Green Light Toolkit in Southampton City, p 18.

Priest H, Gibbs M 2004 Policy issues and service provision. In: Priest H, Gibbs M (eds) Mental health care for people with learning disabilities. Churchill Livingstone, Edinburgh, p 152.

Raghavan R, Patel P 2005 Introduction. In: Raghavan R, Patel P (eds) Learning disabilities and mental health: a nursing perspective. Blackwell Publishing, p 1.

Repper J, Perkins R 2003 Facilitating personal adaptation: taking back control. In: Repper J, Perkins S (eds) Social inclusion and recovery: a model for mental health practice. Bailliere Tindall, p 129.

Scior K, Lango S 2005 In-patient psychiatric care: what can we learn from people with learning disabilities and their carers. Learning Disability Review 10(3):22-23.

Social Services Inspectorate 1998 Moving into the mainstream: an inspection of services for adults with learning disabilities. A summary report for front-line staff and their managers. HMSO, London.

Taggart L, Slevin E 2006 Care planning in mental health settings. In: Gates B (ed) Care planning and delivery in intellectual disability nursing. Blackwell Publishing, p 161-162.

Xenitidis K, Gratsa A, Bouras N et al 2004 Psychiatric inpatient care for adults with intellectual disabilities: generic or specialist units? Journal of Intellectual Disability Research 48(1):11-18.

Intellectual disabilities with mental health problems

Let's be patient: hospital admissions

Rick Robson and Ricky Owens

INTRODUCTION

The aim of this chapter is to identify some of the difficulties that are faced b people with intellectual disabilities, their carers and staff in the acute general hospital; and offer suggestions as to how they might be overcome.

Mainstream health services must be accessible to people with intellectual disabilities. Many people with intellectual disabilities (and their carers) experience episodes of care that are not seen as positive experiences during their stay in the general hospital. The National Patient Safety Agency (2004) identified an admission to the acute hospital as one of their five key areas of concern. The Mencap report 'Death by Indifference' (2007) has stimulated discussion at the highest level; resulting in a Formal Inquiry being ordered by the Secretary of State for Health (2007).

Valuing People (Department of Health 2001) has clearly stated that people with a learning disability must be enabled to access mainstream services:

> 'To enable people with learning disability to access a health service
> designed around their individual needs with fast and convenient care
> delivery to a consistent high standard and with additional support
> when necessary.'
>
> Department of Health 2001

Mainstream health services must therefore be accessible to people with intellectual disabilities.

One of the philosophies behind Valuing People is that there is 'Nothing about us, without us'. For too long now people with intellectual disabilities have had 'things' done to them without any consideration or consultation. It is therefore imperative that people are treated equally when in hospital and that they are treated in an age appropriate manner; particularly in the area of consent.

Concerns have surrounded this area of health care delivery and people with intellectual disabilities for a number of years now. The Department of Health commissioned Cumella & Martin (2000) to examine areas of good practice across the country. This was a small scale study that undertook three workshops across England. What became clearly evident from this work was that there were no national standards or approaches to meet the needs of people with intellectual disabilities (Cumella & Martin 2000).

With advances in medical care, life expectancy for people with intellectual disabilities is approaching that of the general population. Consequently, morbidity and mortality patterns from the general population are beginning to be reflected in people with intellectual disabilities (Barr 1997).

Although this was written over 10 years ago, in fact many people are living longer now and therefore experiencing diseases associated with older age.

Severe intellectual disability is often accompanied by multiple physical disabilities and medical conditions and there are recognised disease associations (e.g. Down's syndrome and Alzheimer's disease). Policy documents emphasise that the health needs of people with intellectual disabilities should be met by mainstream health services, and highlight focal areas where they do not have the same support from, or access to, mainstream health services as the general population (Department of Health 1998, 2001).

The research conducted by Atkinson & Skarloff (1985) (Fig. 7.1) into the care of people with a physical disability identified some damaging areas of concern. The authors suggest that, in fact, little has changed in the intervening years.

The advent of Community Matrons will be an important step forward for the health and well being of each community. These are new posts that have recently been developed following the NHS Improvement Plan (2004) for highly skilled nurses to work with patients who have a high intensity

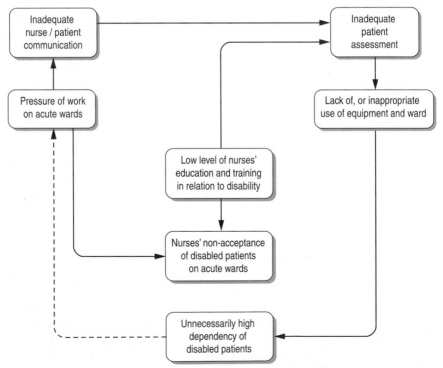

Fig. 7.1 Care of severely disabled people on acute wards (adapted from Atkinson & Skarloff 1985).

of health care support needs such as long term conditions. One of their roles is to prevent frequent admission to hospital. It is necessary for these post holders to understand the health (and associated social) needs of people with an intellectual disability in their local community (Department of Health 2007).

> However the acute hospitals in our area are huge and we do not have the resources or the capacity to work with them because there is no halfway measure. This is such a shame because so many sad stories are still being told about how awful hospital stay is, especially for people with learning disabilities with ageing or complex needs. I have to say it seems to be getting worse and even when we use hospital plans or communication books, they simply don't get read! Even worse are the arguments over funding. LD residential services say they can't afford staff to stay with the person but they are refused extra funding because social services say they are paying for 24-hour care. So a deadlock happens and the person is left stranded in an unfamiliar over stretched environment, with no means of communicating their needs. It scares me it really does! When there is no family, there is no-one or when there is, the family too get no support.
>
> Community Nurse

IDENTIFICATION OF PEOPLE WITH INTELLECTUAL DISABILITIES

One of the difficulties associated with the identification of people with an intellectual disability in a given locality is that data and information are not always shared across agencies. Not all Local Authorities will have a Special Needs Register (SNR) and those that do in many cases only keep a record of the individuals that receive a service. If information sources that do exist are not pulled together, few opportunities exist to gain a detailed picture of local populations.

The NHS has a system for data collection using clinical terms known as 'Read Codes', the aim being to identify patient numbers through their disease or illness type. Unfortunately there are several codes relating to intellectual disability being used across primary care. It is worth noting that these codes only refer to primary care not hospital services.

The plethora of Read Codes being used to identify population groups such as people with intellectual disabilities and the incompatible data collection systems across services can constrain the sharing of information. While acknowledging the purpose of the Data Protection Act (1998) this can potentially lead to an incomplete service.

The increased health needs of the learning disability population is well documented (Mencap 2004). However, the rates of admission for people with intellectual disabilities to hospital are not known. Through the research into attitudes of nursing and medical staff to people with an intellectual disability it might be assumed that not many people are actually admitted (Hart 1998). Prior to the closure of the long stay hospitals, such institutions would have catered for the majority of health needs.

ADMISSION RATES

Morgan et al (2000) identified in their study of patients with an intellectual disability admitted to hospitals in West Glamorgan during the period of 1991–97 that people with an intellectual disability were more likely to have a shorter stay in hospital (4.37 days versus 4.94 days) than the general population. Furthermore that those people with an intellectual disability who lived within institutional settings would be experiencing a much shorter stay than those people who had been discharged into the community (2.1 days versus 5.3 days).

Although patients are classified on admission to hospital, it is only the primary diagnosis and reason for admission that is captured. Hence the 'intellectual disability' as a condition in its own right does not become included with the data. There have been isolated examples of where this information has been collected; sometimes through the Acute Liaison Nurse (see later on in chapter for role clarification) as part of the evaluation of their practice. One of the authors was awaiting an appointment in a local hospital and during a period of 45 minutes observation in a busy outpatients department had earmarked six people as potentially being users of intellectual disability services; multiplying this number across the year gives a very significant number of contacts. Although this was simply an observation and not clinical research or audit it nevertheless implies that a considerable number of people with intellectual disabilities may access the hospital than was previously considered.

THE KNOWLEDGE BASE OF ACUTE CARE STAFF

The lack of awareness of the specific needs of the client group can easily result in the staff in the hospital not being in a position to deliver the optimum care that their patients with an intellectual disability require.

Although we should not be asking them to become experts in intellectual disability, it is reasonable to expect acute care staff to apply their expertise in health issues and its management to the benefit of people with an intellectual disability. Their knowledge therefore needs to encompass (to varying degrees for different staff/professional groups):

- The health needs and 'conditions' that are more likely to be of greater prevalence among people with an intellectual disability
- Basic knowledge and understanding about communication, the principles that underline the philosophy of service delivery and care and an understanding of how this might affect their working practices
- Knowledge of the specialist and other supports that are available within the intellectual disability services for them to call upon for additional help and support.

NURSING ATTITUDES AND STAFFING

Shanley & Guest (1995), in their paper on stigmatisation, highlighted that the nurses' own senses of insecurity in not knowing how to cope with an individual with intellectual disabilities may adversely affect their relationship with the patient. This can lead to the patient being avoided as Adult Nurses find themselves unable to ascertain how to communicate with that individual (Shanley & Guest 1995).

Contact with patients with intellectual disabilities by Adult Nursing students has been shown to facilitate more positive attitudes among nursing staff (Murray & Chambers 1991, Slevin & Sines 1996). Surveys of Adult Nursing students with poor attitudes towards people with intellectual disabilities (Slevin & Sines 1996) have demonstrated that this can result in unmet need. Furthermore, stigmatising attitudes among staff can adversely affect health care for people with intellectual disabilities. A number of studies have reported negative attitudes among nursing staff towards people with intellectual disabilities (Fitzsimons & Barr 1997). In an attempt to overcome this barrier, ward teams will need to receive awareness training on the specific needs of their patients who have an intellectual disability. Often problems will occur when behaviours that challenge the 'system' are presented by the patient themselves. This might be for any number of reasons; but many people with an intellectual disability will not comprehend why they are in a bed with a variety of medical pieces of equipment surrounding them. The Acute Liaison Nurse will be in a position to advise on management strategies and offer support to the patient, their carers and ward staff. Hart (1998) refers to patients being sufficiently occupied in order that they do not become bored.

The Acute Liaison Nurse can be instrumental in ensuring that during a planned admission (e.g. dental work) there can be multiple investigations undertaken during a single general anaesthetic. Known as 'care bundling' a patient might have their hearing tested, bloods taken and even chiropody work undertaken while in the operating theatre. This enables minimal distress to the person with an intellectual disability and maximises the time that clinicians have available to their patient. The co-ordination skills needed to enable these procedures to be undertaken are significant and will demonstrate the way that services can work together better and 'smarter' to the benefit of the patient.

This training should ideally be delivered in multi-disciplinary settings and use people with an intellectual disability as co-trainers. Family carers will be another powerful tool to deliver this message; the personal experiences of these individuals can always have a more lasting impression on the audience.

Occupation of patients' day and time is not seen as part of the role of nursing staff on an acute ward; even though there might be allied health professionals involved in the patient's care they too will not appreciate the need for people to be occupied. This aspect of care will be undertaken by carers if they are available; however this might not be at all times.

Even with policy guidance on service provision, stigmatising attitudes among staff can adversely affect health care for people with intellectual disabilities. Fitzsimons & Barr (1997) review a number of studies reporting negative attitudes among nursing staff and Hart (1998) reports that, of 13 accounts by people with intellectual disability of general hospital care, only one described an interaction which gave the impression of a nurse being genuinely caring. The sentiment put forward by this latter study is echoed in the following quote from 'Death by Indifference' report is the statement '. . . neither would the attitudes displayed by healthcare professionals that result in such a level of fear and mistrust that some families feel the need to mount bedside vigils. . .' (Mencap 2007:4).

CONSENT

The issue of consent is of paramount importance to all healthcare professionals. Unless it can be otherwise demonstrated, all adults should be assessed as having the capacity to consent to treatment. However, this is a 'tricky' area in the case of people with intellectual disabilities.

Why do people let you make decisions?
'It's my life and I can make up my own mind. People encourage me to make decisions for myself; this is part of being treated as an adult. Valuing People says that we have Rights, Independence, Choice and the right to Inclusion.'
What happens when people with learning disabilities go to hospital?
'No one else can make a decision for them; I can make my own and give consent. If people cannot talk then they need to be asked in a different way.'
   Such as?
   'Use accessible information that is user friendly. Use symbols and bigger print – if they can read. Talk to someone else about what is going to happen. The information has got to be shared in good time.'
What are the most important things to remember about consent?
'There has to be easy information. Remember that consent is a complicated issue. Staff have to remain confidential – people wonder what you are writing down. Give people time to understand.'

Ricky Owens 2006

ROLES, RESPONSIBILITIES, EXPECTATIONS

There is often a lack of clarity regarding the roles and responsibilities of professionals and carers, when a person with an intellectual disability is admitted to hospital. Limited protocols exist which outline the responsibility of the hospital.

Paid carers are often in a dilemma as they will have other people for whom they are responsible requiring their time. Staffs in hospital have a different set of expectations to that of carers, which has been expressed through the analogy of 'when the two worlds collide' (Barr 2006). In other words, where the reality of the situation is very differently interpreted by either party. The world of the hospital can be seen as very narrow with little realization of the patients' living circumstances outside the healthy world. The expectation here can lead to differences in how the treatment plans for the patients are delivered. Due to the work pressures in the hospital, staff will not have adequate time to give to a person with an intellectual disability which would meet the satisfaction of most carers.

Staff working in specialist intellectual disability services will generally have a detailed knowledge of the physical illness and the expected course of disorders. Intellectual Disability Nurses will have an intimate knowledge of the client and their individual needs. They should be working collaboratively to share their expertise with acute care staff.

From the hospital staff's perspective, there will obviously be a wide range of cognitive abilities to be considered when assessing each patient, which can lead to confusion regarding the rationale for admission. Ward managers should be able to defend extra staffing for the care of any patient who needs intensive nursing or whose behaviour puts them or others at risk, inadvertently or otherwise. This may demand that family carers/key workers, depending upon the person's living arrangements, are included in the 24-hour care of the patient. This would benefit all parties be it through a reduction in patient anxiety levels (and their carers), the inclusion of carers, in the daily routines and possibly in escorting the patients to theatre or other investigations. Ensure that bleeps and badges are available so that the carers have an identity and are able to take breaks away from the bedside without worry. Slevin & Sines (1996) identified that general nurses valued a carer's presence on the ward as a means of reducing the need for them to become involved with the patient, rather than as an equal member of the team.

Any pre-admission visit will ensure that any of the special nursing needs for people should have become apparent. For some of the people with intellectual disabilities, the initial assessment clearly addressed potential problems and led to appropriate care plans being developed.

Keeping people with intellectual disabilities sedated throughout admission is discriminating and increases the risk of, for example, respiratory infections or pressure sores, to which this group of less mobile patients is already susceptible.

USERS' EXPERIENCES

Some people may identify with previous admissions, others with knowledge gained from watching television programmes and videos, or through talking to friends and carers. Figure 7.2 is a guide to how the Health Service works.

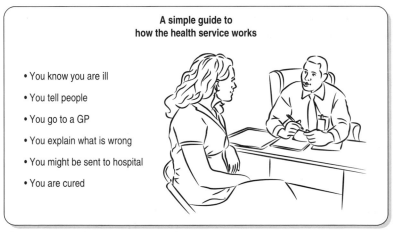

A simple guide to how the health service works

- You know you are ill
- You tell people
- You go to a GP
- You explain what is wrong
- You might be sent to hospital
- You are cured

Fig. 7.2 A simple guide to how the Health Service works.

When seeking views from people with an intellectual disability through face to face interviews and focus groups there was one clear message that came through strongly on each occasion:

'Speak to me, not my carer.'

'Pay more attention to me, not my disability' was another.

The message is that healthcare professionals must engage in a more meaningful manner with their 'patient'.

Time in hospital

- I was anxious because I had not been in the hospital before.
- My temperature increased as I was anxious.
- They were worried in case I had a fit.
- Menu – I told them what I wanted as I can't read all that well.
- Length of fasting – why?
- Tell me what you are doing.
- Too much waiting.
- The Triage Nurse talked to the advocate.
- Simple procedure, long wait.
- Pain was not treated well.
- Signposts need to be improved.
- The doctors and nurses need to communicate more with the patient.

Taking Part Focus Group

This involves information being presented in an accessible format (Easy Read) with careful consideration given to the needs of the individual. This could range from the matters that affect the person most immediately, such as the daily menu sheet, to the consent form being presented in a manner that is understandable. If we are to empower people they have to be in a position to make informed decisions. This can only occur when the information is presented in an easily understood way that enables a choice to be made with the option of having advice given by their supporters.

For any person, an admission to hospital is a worrying time with a great deal of uncertainty and anxiety prevailing. Clearly, information shared with the patient will ease these feelings. When people are stressed it is not unusual for their temperature to rise; this in itself could be misinterpreted by the staff and treated inappropriately. Menu choices were a problem for all of the people with intellectual disabilities and selections can often be made by relatives, staff or other patients. One parent related the events of a prior admission where her son had received no food for 3 days, having made no menu selections because he was unable to read or write. Although six people could feed themselves when well, only two did so when ill. As Hart (1998) also found, the preselection of menu choices proved a problem for all the people with intellectual disabilities in this study, only one of whom could read. An alternative presentation of menu items, such as pictures, would be helpful for those who are able to make choices but have poor understanding of written or spoken language.

Toileting proves problematic for some people with intellectual disabilities, particularly for those people with a pre-existing problem. Where people's continence is supported through the use of continence pads if the ward does not have a supply of these pads then it is likely that the result will be a wet bed and embarrassment. It must be remembered that people do not choose to be incontinent and that there is no fault attached to this outcome.

FAMILY CARERS

Family carers will support their relatives in a way that is often with little or no regard to themselves, being altruistic. Their expectations will, however, be that their relatives are being offered the best possible treatment; and that they will make a full recovery in the shortest possible time.

In this age of information, staff will find that carers are often very knowledgeable about the conditions that are ailing their relatives.

There are too many examples of family carers 'camping' at the bedside due to a lack of confidence in the hospital teams. This may be due to a reluctance to surrender care to others, an acknowledgement that the person will respond best to a carer who knows how to deal with them, or provision of activity for the carer during the day, but there was a generally reported feeling of obligation to help busy staff. Most (family) carers will want to be involved in all aspects of care that is being delivered. Dewing (1991) identified that this might not always be the case where family roles are taken in a more traditional fashion of the mother undertaking the caring role. Responding to different cultural needs is also important.

During longer admissions, it has been the case that many misunderstandings between carers and hospital staff diminish, indicating that problems are related to those of unfamiliarity with people with intellectual disabilities.

Many family carers will wish to stay overnight, but most will not be offered a bed and will end up in bedside chairs. Ward staff will have to be mindful of the emotional effort that families and carers will put into supporting their relative while they are ill.

One of the interventions that was undertaken by the Health Access Nurse was to arrange a series of short visits to the local hospitals for family carers in order that they could see for themselves what the actual wards and environment was all about; prior to the admission. This exercise dispelled a whole range of myths and identified potential problems for each individual carer which they could address in a less hasty manner.

The areas visited included:

The philosophy outlined in 'Valuing People' of working, in collaboration with other colleagues, towards open and easy access to secondary care health

- Medical Emergency Centre
- Head and Neck Unit
- Day Surgery
- Endoscopy
- A & E

- 'Great insight into the areas.'
- 'Staff listened to us and want to work with carers.'
- 'I felt reassured and comfortable that my brothers will be treated with dignity.'
- 'The links with PALS is great.'
- 'Thank you for reassuring me that my son would be well looked after.'
- 'Recognition by the Trust that people need to know what goes on in hospital is a great step forward.'

Family carers' comments

services for people with an intellectual disability will scope the role 'allow the role to extend' of the Acute Liaison Nurse.

As the workload within the general hospital has altered dramatically with a greater emphasis on a rapid turnover of patients and more access to care near or at home (Our Health, Our Care, Our Say; Department of Health 2006). Many of the problems faced by people with an intellectual disability, their carers and staff can be addressed by the intervention of the Acute Liaison Nurse; a person whose brief it is to have the time to be proactive in the planning of any admission and/or the support the wards in the cases of emergencies.

These positions are invaluable in demonstrating nursing skills at their highest level as the nurse becomes recognised for their knowledge and skill in dealing with individual issues. For the role to be successful, achieving small successes is essential both for the department and through engaging with staff to gain the best possible care. This might be through the Essence of Care work, which would clearly be endorsed by the Director of Nursing at the hospital. A useful task to undertake is a guide to the staff in the hospital through identification of staff uniforms. While there are some common colours used for some staff groups – Physiotherapists in Blue and Occupational Therapists in Green – these might not always be the case and add to the confusion.

There are many examples of the positive interventions undertaken by Acute Liaison Nurses across the UK. With the National A2A (Access to Acutes) network being an excellent way of disseminating good practice, particularly relevant where nurses have been seconded into these roles as project workers. Some of the key functions in their job descriptions might include:

- To raise the profile of the health care needs of people with an intellectual disability across secondary care provision.
- To bridge the gap between intellectual disability and secondary services to enable better communication and access to healthcare for people with intellectual disabilities.
- To assess and advise accordingly on the issues surrounding the complex needs of some people with intellectual disabilities, on their admission to hospital care settings.
- To work in partnership with people with intellectual disabilities, self advocacy group, PALS and carers' groups in the development, implementation and maintenance of service provision.
- To develop and maintain networking and liaison with partners in primary, community and intellectual disability services.

- To assist in the development of local strategies and minimum standards for working with people with intellectual disabilities when in hospital.
- To coordinate and assist in the delivery of training to meet identified needs specifically to ensure that colleagues in acute hospitals are aware of and able to meet the needs of people with an intellectual disability.

PAIN AND DISCOMFORT

It will always be an area where healthcare staff can make a significant difference to the lives and experiences of people with intellectual disabilities. Table 7.1 and Figure 7.3 identify some of the features that people might present when they are in pain or discomfort. Hospital staff and carers must learn to observe whether pain is being experienced, particularly by those people who are non-verbal. If in doubt it is the duty of care to administer analgesia.

The beauty of using the picture in Figure 7.3 is that the patient can be involved in their own assessment of their pain. All too often the nurses will rush by during the medicines round and quickly ask 'Everything OK?' Where there is no answer, this could be interpreted as 'no pain' and therefore no pain relief would be administered. Nursing staff can use the numerical scoring system to record the subjective pain reported by patients. All that is required is a person-centred approach to care and using the assessment skills and knowledge base to determine the comfort or discomfort levels of the person who is unable to self report.

IF YOU DON'T KNOW WHAT TO ASK FOR THEN HOW CAN YOU ASK FOR HELP?

Table 7.1   Signs and symptoms of pain or discomfort

Facial expressions	Verbalisations	Vocalisations
Grimacing	Self reports	Sighing
Specific	Complaining	Crying
Configurations of	Asking for help	Moaning
fear	Repeated requests	Groaning
Sadness	for analgesia	Other non-language
Disgust		sounds

1   2   3   4   5

Fig. 7.3   The faces of pain.

RECOMMENDATIONS TO REDUCE HEALTH INEQUALITIES IN ACUTE CARE

- Action to reduce health inequalities: to explore the feasibility of establishing a confidential inquiry into mortality among people with intellectual disabilities
- Action to challenge discrimination against people with intellectual disabilities from minority ethnic communities

People with intellectual disabilities and their carers frequently express concerns about the attitudes and treatment they experience when using general hospital outpatient, A&E or inpatient services. Recommendations include:

- Training of staff by patients
- Introductory visits
- Videos of the hospital: Sec 4.26.

Signposts for Success Department of Health 1998

A2A – ACCESS TO ACUTES

In the light of experience and dissatisfaction with the service that many people received, the authors established the A2A Network in 1999.

This network now has a growing membership, principally of Intellectual Disability Nurses, but with other interested parties as well. There are quarterly national meetings and now regional groups have been formed to ensure that there is a wider involvement. More information is available at www.nnldn.org/a2a. These form excellent opportunities for individuals to share good practice and network; the results can clearly be seen as work is translated across the country.

BETTER METRICS NO. 11

These standards were described by the Strategic Health Authority in 2005, and yet to date they have not been monitored effectively. This has resulted in yet another opportunity being lost for services to people with an intellectual disability and their families to be improved.

Objective: To ensure that people with intellectual disability are appropriately supported during acute care.

Metric: Acute hospitals have a system in place to ensure that people with intellectual disability are identified and appropriate support is provided.

As is apparent from the reader's own knowledge of these subject matters, the implemention of an effective method of capturing accurate numbers of people who use the services of their local hospital would ensure that a better understanding of the issues would assist in reducing the problems faced by people and their families/carers.

INTELLECTUAL DISABILITY AND SOCIAL INCLUSION

Following their 'Treat me Right' (2004) campaign, Mencap have taken the experiences of six families who had poor experiences while their family members were in the care of the local General Hospital. While these six accounts are of people who died unnecessarily, there have been many others who have too had an early death as a result of inappropriate treatment. The Secretary of State for Health instructed that an Independent National Inquiry should be held and the six cases were also referred to the Health Service Ombudsman. The reports are awaited as of May 2008.

Mencap identified six key issues in their report that they are calling for further action to be taken on:

- People with intellectual disabilities are seen as a low priority.
- Many healthcare professionals do not understand much about intellectual disabilities.
- Many healthcare professionals do not properly consult and involve the families and carers of people with intellectual disabilities.
- Many healthcare professionals do not understand the law around capacity and consent to treatment.
- Healthcare professionals rely inappropriately on their estimates of the person's quality of life.
- The complaints system within the NHS services is often ineffectual, time consuming and inaccessible.

'Death by Indifference' (Mencap 2007)

Recommendations from the Mencap Report

- Clearer identification of the needs of a person prior to their admission. This could be through improved letters of referral from GPs and other practitioners.
- Listen carefully to the carers; they will have vast experience of the person's needs – particularly family carers.
- Support for family carers and paid carers who need to accompany the person through their stay in hospital.
- Simple measures such as free meals, car parking, accommodation nearby the patient, badges identifying the person as a 'Carer'.
- A system of identifying people on their case notes, electronic records or data bases that additional support needs were required for these patients to have a successful admission to hospital.
- To improve the training and awareness raising of all staff working within the hospital to ensure that all vulnerable people were supported according to their needs.
- Discuss with Commissioners and Lead Nurses.
- Ask again.

Recommendations from carers

- Listen carefully to the carers; they will have vast experience of the person's needs – particularly family carers.

Let's be patient: hospital admissions

- Support for family carers and paid carers who need to accompany the person through their stay in hospital.
- Simple measures such as free meals, car parking, accommodation nearby the patient, badges identifying the person as a 'Carer'.
- A system of identifying people on their case notes, electronic records or data bases that additional support needs were required for these patients to have a successful admission to hospital.
- To improve the training and awareness raising of all staff working within the hospital to ensure that all vulnerable people were supported according to their needs.

Recommendations for people with an intellectual disability

- Use pre-admission visits for routine admissions.
- Explain to the patient what is happening now and next using accessible communication aids.
- Avoid unnecessary sedation and procedures.
- Respond to the person in an age appropriate manner.
- Offer positive experiences with people with intellectual disabilities as part of nurse and doctor training.
- Arrange extra staff when necessary.
- Use a side-room if necessary, otherwise a bed near the nurses' station.

CONCLUSION

Once again, it can be seen that little action has taken place from Government and the NHS and that the discrimination will continue. There will be no new recommendations until the 'old/original' ones are taken forward and embedded within the day to day practice of all healthcare professionals.

'If we can get it right for people with an intellectual disability then we shall get it right for everyone.'

Ricky Owens

REFERENCES

Atkinson F A, Sklaroff S A 1987 Acute hospital wards and the disabled patient. Royal College of Nursing, London.

Barr O 1997 Care of people with learning disabilities in hospital. Nursing Standard 12:49–56.

Barr O 2006 When two worlds collide – a keynote presentation at the Learning Disability Nursing National Forum Conference, 17 November 2006. RCN, London.

Barr O 2006 'When two worlds collide' presentation. In: Royal College of Nursing annual Learning Disabilities conference. London, November 2006.

Cumella S, Martin D 2000 Secondary healthcare for people with a learning disability. Department of Health – unpublished.

Department of Health 1998 Signposts for success in commissioning and providing health services for people with learning disabilities. HMSO, London.

Department of Health 2001 'Valuing People – A strategy for the 21st Century'. HMSO, London.

Department of Health 2006 'Our Health, our care, our say' – a new direction for services. HMSO, London.

Dewing J 1991 Physically disabled people in acute care. Nursing Standard 5:37-39.

Fitzsimons J, Barr O 1997 A review of reported attitudes of health and social care professionals towards people with learning disabilities. Journal of Learning Disabilities, Nursing, Health and Social Care 1(2):57-64.

Fox D, Wilson D 1999 Parents' experiences of general hospital admission for adults with learning disabilities. Journal of Clinical Nursing 8:610-614.

Hart S L 1998 Learning-disabled people's experience of general hospitals. British Journal of Nursing 7:470-477.

Hollins S, Attard M T, von Fraunhofer N, Sedgwick P 1998 Mortality in people with learning disability: risks, causes, and death certification findings in London. Developmental Medicine & Child Neurology 40:50-56.

Lindsey M, Singh K, Perrett A 1993 Management of learning disability in the general hospital. British Journal of Hospital Medicine 50:182-186.

Mason J, Scior K 2004 Diagnostic overshadowing amongst clinicians working with people with intellectual disabilities in the UK. Journal of Applied Research in Intellectual Disabilities 17(2):85-90.

McGuigan S M, Hollins S, Attard M 1995 Age-specific standardized mortality rates in people with learning disability. Journal of Intellectual Disability Research 39:527-531.

Mencap 2004 Treat me right: better healthcare for people with a learning disability. Mencap, London.

Mencap 2007 Death by indifference. Mencap, London.

Morgan C L, Ahmed Z, Kerr M P 2000 Healthcare provision for people with a learning disability. Record-linkage study of epidemiology and factors contributing to hospital care uptake. British Journal of Psychiatry 176(1):37-41.

Murray M, Chambers M 1991 Effect of contact on nursing students' attitudes to patients. Nurse Education Today 11:363-367.

National Patient Safety Agency 2004 Understanding the Patient Safety Issues for people with a learning disability. National Patient Safety Agency NHS, Febuary 2004.

Royal College of Nursing 2006 Meeting the health needs of people with learning disabilities. RCN, London (revised 2007).

Shanley E, Guest C 1995 Stigmatisation of people with learning disabilities in general hospitals. British Journal of Nursing 4(13):759-760.

Slevin E, Sines D 1996 Attitudes of nurses in a general hospital towards people with learning disabilities: influences of contact, and graduate/non-graduate status: a comparative study. Journal of Advanced Nursing 24:1116-1126.

Let's be patient: hospital admissions

Primary care and intellectual disability

Susan Brady and Martin Bollard

INTRODUCTION

Primary care provides the linchpin to health services for adults with intellectual disabilities. Primary care as a model of care delivery should be locally based, responsive and able to deploy resources appropriately to meet the complexity of needs of the patients it serves (Department of Health 1997). People with intellectual disabilities have the same right of access to mainstream services as anyone else, but may require additional support to use them (Disability Rights Commission 2006).

Providing effective primary care for people with intellectual disabilities is a challenge. Despite 12 years of Government initiatives aimed at addressing the inequalities faced by people with intellectual disabilities when accessing primary healthcare (Department of Health 1998, 1999, 2001, 2005) progress has been difficult. Pockets of good practice across the country are evident (Department of Health 2007a, Martin & Martin 2000, Roy & Martin 1999) but there remains misunderstanding around consent processes and people with intellectual disabilities still experiencing many barriers when accessing the health care services that they require.

Specialist Learning Disability Services are the main National Health Service provision for people with intellectual disabilities. The way in which professionals working within these services can support primary health care has been actively promoted over the last decade (Barr et al 1999, Bollard & Jukes 1999, Cumella et al 1992, Department of Health 1999, 2001, 2007). However, ensuring effective access to primary care should be the responsibility of all professionals working within the primary health care sector.

With the political drive to reduce NHS provision for this group of people (Department of Health 2007b), more emphasis will be placed on supporting social care to work alongside people with intellectual disabilities to gain equitable access to primary health care. To adequately meet the generic and specific health needs of this group of people, primary care will require persistent and active support from all stakeholders, if the aspiration of primary care ownership (Department of Health 2001) in relation to people with intellectual disabilities is to be realised.

Health Facilitation is one way that has been suggested could help meet this ideal alongside planning care through the development of Health Action Plans (HAPs) (Department of Health 2001).

This chapter reports on two sets of evaluation based primarily on the experiences of people with intellectual disabilities. The work is drawn from an extensive primary health care project conducted in Birmingham spanning just over 4 years from September 1999 to March 2004. From that work, two sets of data will be presented. Initially the experiences and viewpoints of going to the doctors and secondly how people with intellectual disabilities perceive the work of health facilitators and the utility of Health Action Plans.

BACKGROUND

The Death by Indifference report (Mencap 2007) highlighted that people with intellectual disabilities die unnecessarily. Evidence in the document suggests that certain patients with intellectual disabilities could have got better if they had received the right treatment or care. The poor response by acute care to this group of people, as highlighted through the case studies within the report (Mencap 2007), points to institutional discrimination. Although the report focused on case studies related to acute care, the necessity to promote the rights to equitable health care transcends all mainstream health provision for people with intellectual disabilities.

The possible reasons for this tacit discrimination demonstrated within the report (Mencap 2007) are multi-faceted. Apart from a general lack of understanding of intellectual disabilities within mainstream health services, many health professionals find it difficult to adapt to meet the needs of people with intellectual disabilities (Barr et al 2006). In many cases, health care professionals are not always conversant with the law around capacity and consent that relates to this vulnerable group of people. They require training to understand intellectual disability itself and how to effectively establish an individual's method of communication to gauge their capacity to consent and what support is required to ensure consent is informed. Furthermore in the busy and stretched National Health Service, the reasonable adjustments necessary to meet the needs of this group of people may not be solely down to a lack of training but are due to either subliminal or blatant discrimination.

The Disability Discrimination Act (1995) was established to provide all people with disabilities the protection from discrimination. Since 1st October 1999, service providers have had to take reasonable steps to change practices and procedures that make it unreasonably difficult for disabled people to use a service. The Mental Capacity Act (2005) which came into force in April 2007 makes it clear that all individuals over the age of 16 are presumed to have the capacity and right to make his or her own decisions unless it is proved otherwise. This clearly relates to all forms of health care.

Effective communication is central to any debate about access to health care (Law et al 2005). The shifting emphasis on health decision making away from the health professional to the patient/service user (Department of Health 2001b) demands that individuals can identify and articulate their health needs. Exactly how this can be achieved effectively by people who present with specific communication difficulties within primary care is not yet fully established.

Information given to the disabled person must be in an accessible format taking into consideration the individual's specific communication needs. Research has shown that practical resources such as handbooks, resource guides (Lennox et al 1997), lists of specialist physicians, referral guides and policy documents on informed consent that relate to people with intellectual disabilities (Minihan et al 1993) have all been highlighted as useful by primary care physicians. Therefore the communication of information and ensuring understanding of the implications of different choices are key elements to giving informed consent.

The importance of building up the doctor–patient relationship for people with longstanding and complex medical conditions is important (Lewis & Dixon 2005:12) and all workers should continue to assist this bedrock aspect of primary care practice for all people with intellectual disabilities. Furthermore, the complex symptomology and the common communication difficulties associated with many people with intellectual disabilities makes this group of people vulnerable to 'secondary complexities' (Heyman et al 2004). In order to manage modern health care with finite resources, it is necessary to standardise, rationalise and simplify complex health needs. Such simplified service models do not always suit the needs of people with intellectual disabilities (Heyman et al 2004) and the contribution that all workers can make in order to respond to complexity should not be underestimated for this particular group of people. Health Action Plans mediated through effective health facilitation is one way that can respond to the complexity of needs often presented within primary health care by people with intellectual disabilities.

At the point of access into primary care, many people with intellectual disabilities may well require additional assistance to fully participate and have their needs clearly identified. This can present something of a paradox, as the modern health care system calls for individuals to be empowered (Department of Health 1997, 2001b) and assumes that power is something that can be simply given away by those that have it and readily taken on by those that need it (Zarb 1992). This is naturally not that straightforward for people with intellectual disabilities and significant amounts of time are invested by specialist intellectual disabilities nurses/health facilitators, carers and others to overcome this latter power differential through the provision of accessible health materials and varying methods of support. The intention here is to ensure as best possible, the smooth navigation in and out of the primary care system for people with intellectual disabilities.

In attempts to overcome the access to primary care difficulties, many nurses and workers in the intellectual disability field have sought to work alongside their primary care colleagues. Valuing People (Department of Health 2001) requires both general and specialist services to work together to reduce the health inequalities experienced by people with intellectual disabilities. People with intellectual disabilities should have equal access to the health services they need with additional support to use those services if required. The need for non-specialist health professionals to have adequate skills in communication when providing a health service to people with intellectual disabilities has been well documented (Lindsey 2002, Mencap 2004, Powrie 2003, Scottish Executive 2002, Sperlinger 1997). This is particularly problematic within the area of primary health care, where the general practitioner is reliant on the patient to identify and explain their health needs. Aspray et al (1999) expressed concern that specialist knowledge in intellectual disabilities is not accessible to all health professionals who need it. Through a survey, Minihan et al (1993) highlighted particular problems with informed consent with 53% of physicians reporting that they did not know who was authorised to give consent for medical treatment of their patients with intellectual disabilities, and 65% not knowing where to obtain any further information. A further finding highlighted in this study was that only one in five primary care physicians reported that they felt well prepared to handle a patient with intellectual disabilities, when refusing to cooperate with an examination or treatment (Minihan et al 1993). A study in the UK had similar findings, suggesting that 64% of physicians were unaware of the correct procedures for consent to treatment for people with intellectual disabilities according to English law (Turner et al 1999).

The recent report Closing the Gap: Equal Treatment by the Disability Rights Commission (2006) has stated that people with intellectual disabilities receive fewer screening tests and fewer health investigations then the general population. This has implications for morbidity and mortality of the intellectual disability population. Box 8.1 contains a summary of the report.

Box 8.1   Key Disability Rights Commission (2006) report findings

Intellectual disability not seen as priority

People with intellectual disability are not always offered treatment options that are offered to the rest of the population

Around 30% primary care practitioners believe that the health care needs of people with intellectual disability are provided and monitored by specialist services

Routine annual health screening is patchy

Assumptions are made about health treatment options without consultation with adults who have intellectual disability

National Service Frameworks overlook the specific needs/requirements of people with intellectual disability

People who exhibit challenging behaviour are seen less frequently by their GP than the rest of the intellectual disability population

Communication barriers between primary care professionals and people with intellectual disability

High levels of referrals to primary care are not managed appropriately/effectively

Issues with consent to treatment/rights of adults with intellectual disability are overlooked.

GPs in inner city areas have increased case loads

Accessible information/health promotion is not readily available in all primary care establishments

Ways of assisting general practice – Health Facilitation and HAPs

There are multi-faceted reasons why achieving good primary care for people with intellectual disabilities is a challenge. Some of this literature on communication and consent has already been highlighted as one pivotal aspect.

> 'Integration of people with a learning disability into a primary care system . . . will not occur by relying on generic primary health care services to develop this in isolation.'
>
> Rodgers 1993:22

Collaboration between primary, secondary and acute services has been suggested as the way forward to promote better services (Brady et al 2002, Glasby 2002, Martin et al 1999). Historically, specialist intellectual disability services have provided an all encompassing service meeting the generic and specific needs of this group of people. In some cases this has not allowed general practice to develop its ownership and ability to recognise and meet the health needs of people with intellectual disabilities.

The role of health facilitation in intellectual disabilities has been advocated as one way in which specialist intellectual disability nurses and others can bridge the gap between secondary care (specialist services) and primary and acute care (Department of Health 2001).

Supporting annual health checks for people with intellectual disabilities

All community nurses working within Birmingham are supporting people with intellectual disabilities known to the intellectual disability service to access an annual health check and health action plan. Those additional people with intellectual disabilities that do not currently receive a service are being supported by identified health facilitators for the PCT area in conjunction with their own GP practice. An evidence based health screening template is available to all practices to enable them to provide a suitable annual health check for people with intellectual disabilities that addresses their specific health needs. Accessible appointment letters and materials have been produced by the health facilitators to support the health check. A primary care guidance sheet for the health check has also been produced to assist with communication barriers that exist between people with an intellectual disability and their primary care team. The health facilitators focus on particular barriers to accessing the health check and work with the person with an intellectual disability, their carers and the primary care team to overcome them.

Unmet health needs of people with intellectual disabilities

Hatton et al (2003) highlighted that people with intellectual disabilities are more likely to suffer from certain conditions as shown in Box 8.2 than the rest of the population:

Despite these high levels of associated health problems shown in Box 8.2, improvements in medical screening and treatment has meant that people with intellectual disabilities are now living longer (Puri et al 1995). However, they still

Box 8.2   Specific health needs of people with intellectual
disabilities

Cancer	Dementia
Coronary heart disease	Osteoporosis
Respiratory disease	Poor oral health
Epilepsy	Thyroid dysfunction
Sensory impairments	Mental health

remain at high risk of an early death compared to the rest of the population (Hollins et al 1998, McGuigan et al 1995). The 'Death by Indifference' report by Mencap (2007) highlighted the preventable deaths of a number of people with intellectual disabilities, demonstrating examples of poor healthcare that this group of people can experience. People with Down's syndrome are particularly at risk of physical complications as a result of their syndrome (Prasher 1995). Individuals with respiratory disease and dysphagia are also at greater risk. Respiratory disease is reported to be the leading cause of death in people with intellectual disabilities (Carter & Jancar 1993). Hollins et al (1998) and Puri et al (1995) reported incidents being much greater than the rest of the general population.

Communication barriers with patients and other health professionals along with problems obtaining patient histories are highlighted as the two most significant barriers to effective healthcare for people with intellectual disabilities (Lennox et al 1997). To add to this problem there is evidence to suggest that carers and other health care professionals find it difficult to recognise the health needs of people with intellectual disabilities (Harries 1991, Howells 1986). Kerins et al (2004) found that primary care physicians believed that caring for people with intellectual disabilities was more difficult compared to other groups. This was attributed to lack of education and training pertaining to patients with intellectual disabilities, issues of communication and interruptions in the continuity of patient care.

In a study conducted by Thornton (1999), the general practitioner (GP) was seen to be the co-ordinator of health care for people with intellectual disabilities. However the participants in the study questioned their effectiveness in relation to their own experiences of accessing health care services. Many identified the Learning Disability Nurse to be the key co-ordinator of their healthcare. It is important therefore that these experiences of both providing and receiving healthcare are communicated effectively to all those involved.

METHODOLOGY

Qualitative research combines the scientific and artistic natures of nursing to enhance understanding of the human health experience (LoBiondo-Wood & Haber 2002). This research approach was considered appropriate to underpin these evaluations as it focuses on the experiences of the service users in this context of primary care. It is acknowledged that involving people with intellectual disabilities in research can be fraught with challenges (Kiernan 1999). Yet nowadays more and more ways of involving people with intellectual disabilities in the traditional aspects of the research process are being found (Walmsley & Johnson 2003).

Qualitative studies can be used as part of service development or service evaluation which can provide a platform to engage individuals that are already receiving a health care service (LoBiondo-Wood & Haber 2002). However ethical considerations are always of paramount importance when involving humans in the research process. The consent process to take part in the evaluation was assisted by preparatory work undertaken by the project lead (Susan Brady). The service users were further informed about the evaluation by encompassing focus groups, semi structured interviews and accessible questionnaires with service users already known to the Health Facilitation Team in Birmingham. Qualitative research has been utilised in both evaluative studies in Birmingham. This research approach focuses on the human experience (Bryman 2004) of working with Health Facilitators and receiving a Health Action Plan.

In order to ensure that any future service development encompassed the views of service users the project lead approached two local day centres in Birmingham one in the north and one in the south. The project lead spoke to the day centre managers to seek permission to conduct 1:1 interviews with service users and their carers and also to hold a focus group meeting on the premises. Initially a standard accessible letter was drafted and sent out to service users and their families that attended the day centres. The project Lead also met with individuals who attended the day centres to talk about healthy lifestyles and health promotion issues. These were weekly sessions facilitated by the project lead. This was done to encourage individuals to think about their health and to understand their rights within the health care environment. The project lead felt that by familiarising herself with the participants it would encourage them to feel more comfortable about sharing their views and experiences. 1:1 interviews utilising semi-structured questionnaires that were completed by the project lead were conducted over a 6-month period. The questionnaire was approved by a multi- professional panel prior to implementation. The analysis was not able to select individual comments from the service users or the carers. The responses are therefore presented as a collective dialogue generated between the service users and the carers that was facilitated by the project lead.

FINDINGS

Service users/carers perspective of going to the doctors

Prior to the offer of an annual health check and health action plan a total of 203 service users and their carers were identified to participate in semi-structured 1:1 interviews with the project lead to comment on their experiences of accessing primary care services. The findings are collective responses from both service users and carers.

The service users reported their attendance at their doctors over the last 12 months, 6 months, month or a week: Most attended within a month:

- Reported attending within a week (21%)
- Within a month (28%)
- Within 6 months (14%)
- Within 12 months (14%)
- Didn't know (23%)

The service users and carers reported favourably on the experience of going to the doctors:

Liked going (78%)
- Disliked going (14%)
- Undecided (8%)

The service users and carers were then asked the following questions:

What are the good things about going to the doctors?
Company and attention; the doctor is alright he smiles and has a joke;
the doctor is nice he listens to you; having my immunisations to stop me getting ill;
helped me understand about my periods which has stopped me worrying
It's OK to go to the doctors. He asks me how I am and he cares about me
My doctor is nice. He talks to me and makes me less nervous.

What worries you most when you are unwell and have to see the doctor or go to hospital?
Waiting for my turn to see the doctor
Don't like too many people in the surgery
Getting to the surgery
Long waiting times
Impatience of primary care staff
Inconvenient appointments
Lack of accessible premises
Support to get service user to the premises
Lack of advocacy support
Barriers to communication
Knowing when to say I am in pain
Being informed about treatment plan and outcome
Issues around consent to treatment
Service user views being ignored
Assumptions being made about the person because they have an L/D
Lack of appropriate screening opportunities
Services that are offered being inappropriate to meet the needs of the service user

What support do you need when going to the doctors?
Information leaflets that I can understand
Regular check-ups
Help to order my tablets
Two staff to support me to get to the surgery
I don't always tell the doctor the truth about how I am feeling
I need to be persuaded to go to the doctors and hospital because I feel there is nothing wrong with me
Health staff that speak my language
I want someone to explain to me how I can stay healthy in a way I understand
Would like to be seen at home
Staff to talk slower
Appointments to fit around college and Day Centre because of my transport arrangements

FINDINGS

The following findings relate to the experiences of the service users in relation to health facilitation and health action planning. The focus group was established to report on the experiences of six service users attending a local day centre. Three were male and three were female; their ages ranged from 20 to 62 years. One meeting was arranged with service users. The discussions held during the focus group meeting have been analysed using content analysis (May 2007) and the following themes were elicited:

Reassurance and support

I was worried about having my blood taken but the nurse helped me not to worry. She told me what was going to happen. I wasn't able to get to the doctors on my own so the Health Facilitator arranged for someone to come to see me at home.

I like the Health Action Planning pack. It's all about me.

Jackie said that when she went into hospital she had a special plan that gave information about all her tests and treatment. It had writing and pictures in it.

The plan was given to her family as well. Jackie said this helped her a lot. It stopped her feeling so worried about being in hospital.

Practical assistance

Health Facilitator helped me arrange appointments.

I couldn't walk because my toe nails were digging in under my feet. I didn't know who to ask about it. The Health Facilitator arranged for a man to make my feet better. He came to see me at home to cut my nails. He visits me every 3 months at home because I can't find my way to the doctors.

The nurse helped me to stop smoking.

I love my hand held record. It is just like a diary of all my needs.

I went to the doctors for my health check and found that I had lots of things wrong with me. Now everyone is helping to make me feel better.

Education

I didn't understand the information leaflets. The Health Facilitators made me a plan that had pictures so that I knew what I had to do to stay healthy.

The Health Facilitator chatted to me about my health and what I needed to do to stay healthy.

I can't read. The Health Facilitator gave me leaflets with pictures about my health.

The Health Facilitator showed our group home how to examine our breasts for lumps. I am frightened about getting cancer like my mom had. The Health Facilitator stopped me worrying and told me what I needed to do.

I have diabetes. The Health Facilitator showed me how to check my blood and what to do if I felt poorly.

At our meeting the nurses told us all about Health Action Plans and Health Facilitation. Some of us had heard about it like Jackie, but most of us didn't know what it meant.

Empowerment

The focus group helped us to say what we thought was important and what we needed to do to stay healthy. It was easier to talk in a small group. We had a green card which we held in the air if we had something to say and a red card if we didn't agree with something. This was to help people who didn't like to speak up as much.

Continued

Empowerment—cont'd

The resource pack was produced to help us make our own Health Action Plans. The group talked about some of their own health problems like diabetes, high blood pressure, high cholesterol and epilepsy. We told each other how we usually look after our own health. We were given a choice about how we wanted our Health Action Plan to be made.

Some of the things the service users felt were important to help them take care of their health problems were:

- A contact card
- Contact person (like a nurse)
- Other professionals involved
- Some of us liked to use a hand held record or plan
- Everyone has a communication book which is good

We looked at different ways that our Health Action Plans could be made:

- Photographs
- Pictures and symbols
- Written
- Tapes
- Accessible leaflets

We liked the idea of the communication books and photographs for our Health Action Plans best because they were more personal to us. We asked if the communication books could be made smaller and in different colours so that we could have more choice. Some people needed them in different languages.

DISCUSSION

In many ways the experience drawn from the users and carers of going to the doctors is similar to that of other vulnerable groups of people. Getting to the doctors and waiting can be difficult for all people with disabilities. What this engagement with users and carers has shown is that professional support, assistance and the production of accessible Health Action Plans that are tailored to meet individual need is valued by users.

The consultation process highlighted in the Birmingham project has been essential to ensure that service user/carer views and experiences were heard and acted upon. This has a wider relevance as little is known about the benefit of Health Facilitation and Health Action Plans from the user and carer perspective.

Communication difficulties have been highlighted as a key barrier for people with intellectual disabilities being offered and receiving appropriate health care services (Lennox et al 1997). Promoting communication for individuals with intellectual disabilities and primary care staff has formed an integral part of the health facilitation development process in Birmingham.

Following the guidance that has been available on Health Action Planning, GP practices across Birmingham are now actively working in partnership with the Health Facilitators to offer Health Action Plans to their patients with an intellectual disability. The specific risk factors identified as part of an individual's annual health check form the basis for an individual's

Health Action Plan. Health Facilitators and Community Nurses are completing Health Action Plans in accessible formats in collaboration with primary care services for all people with intellectual disabilities identified on practice lists. This work has been a key plank to achieving the necessary improvements in the health of people with intellectual disabilities (Department of Health 2007b).

Support and information is also being issued to individuals with an intellectual disability, their carers and residential homes to enable them to facilitate a Health Action Plan for the people they care for. This type of practical assistance and education was a key theme that came from the focus group with the users. Any plans that are produced are being recorded on the intellectual disability health screening template within GP practices so that appropriate referrals and reviews can be actioned or monitored as required. Establishing this type of system to monitor health needs for people with intellectual disabilities is essential, if improvements in primary care for people with intellectual disabilities are going to be sustained.

What is evident from available research is that in order to improve communication between providers of healthcare and the individual with intellectual disabilities there needs to be an effective interface. Appropriate support for people with intellectual disabilities requires face to face meetings between clinician and patient so that both can learn from each other (Martin 2005). Accessible information and good communication skills are crucial if people with intellectual disabilities are to have equal access to both primary and secondary health care. Individuals need to be able to access information they can understand and with which they can make decisions about their health (Royal College of Nursing 2006).

In the past it was assumed that having an intellectual disability meant people lacked capacity to make decisions (Royal College of Nursing 2006). However, it is now recognised that the UK laws on consent to examination and treatment serve the whole population including those with intellectual disabilities (Department of Health 2005, Scottish Executive 2000). Now more than ever people with intellectual disabilities are in a 'position to have their say'. It is important to recognise the equal importance of 'empowerment'. Although the sample of users was small in the second study reported in this chapter, empowerment was a key theme elicited from the focus group with the users.

By keeping the individual with intellectual disability informed prior to and during any healthcare experience their experiences can be improved considerably (Brady et al 2002). Definitions on empowerment are wide-ranging and have not been adequately defined (Kuokkanen et al 2000). What is known is that it is concerned with '*power, authority and facilitation*' which in turn can lead to improved quality of intervention and better processes associated with the individual and their environment. Empowerment can be seen as the opportunity to take action, the outcome being the generation of positive results at both an individual and organisational level. Thomas & Velthouse (1990) described it as a process of personal growth and development in which key factors are the individual's characteristics such as '*beliefs, views, values, perceptions and relationships*' with the environment. Empowerment and operating in a person centred way should be a central focus to practitioners facilitating health and developing Health Action Plans within primary care.

CONCLUDING COMMENTS

By focusing on the views and experiences of people with intellectual disabilities a better understanding of what is 'real' promotes guidance for nursing practice. By empowering individuals and their carers, communication barriers can be addressed which in turn could lead to better health outcomes for people with intellectual disabilities. Health Action Planning goes hand in hand with Health Facilitation. By establishing an effective system for joint health screening, which is supported by health facilitators, a Health Action Planning Process can be established and monitored. This can be done by continuing to educate and support primary care, service users and their carers around issues concerned with health needs, risks, planning of care and health promotion.

If effective links and partnership working is maintained with primary care across all PCT areas in Birmingham, the Learning Disability Service should be able to meet the Government's targets for meeting the health needs of people with intellectual disabilities. In order for this to occur, specialist community staff, not just nurses, need to examine their current roles to incorporate health facilitation. Alternatively specialised health facilitators who are providing dedicated time, training and resources to support primary care directly may also guide the way forward.

REFERENCES

Aspray T, Francis R M, Tyler S P, Quillam S J 1999 Patients with learning disability in the community. British Medical Journal 318:476-477.

Barr O, Gilgunn J, Kane T, Moore G 1999 Health screening for people with learning disabilities by a community nursing service in Northern Ireland. Journal of Advanced Nursing 29(6):1482-1491.

Barr O 2006 'When two worlds collide'. Keynote presentation, Learning Disability National Forum Conference, 17 September 2006. RCN, London.

Bollard M, Jukes M J D 1999 Specialist practitioner within community learning disabilities and the primary health care team. Journal of Learning Disabilities 3(1):11-19.

Brady S, Ahmad F, Bissaker S 2002 Partnership for Developing Quality care pathway initiative for people with learning disabilities. Journal of Integrated Care Pathways 6:82-85.

Bryman A 2004 Social research methods. Oxford University Press.

Carter G, Jancar J 1983 Mortality in the mentally handicapped: a 50 year survey at Stoke Park group of hospitals (1930–1980). Journal of Mental Deficiency Research 27:143-156.

Cumella et al 1992 Primary Health Care for people with learning disability. Mental Handicap 201:123-125.

Department of Health 1995 The Health of the nation. HMSO, London.

Department of Health 1997 The NHS modern. Dependable. Department of Health, London.

Department of Health 1998 Signposts for success in commissioning and providing health services for people with learning disabilities. NHS Executive, London.

Department of Health 1999 Once a Day. NHS Executive, London.

Department of Health 2001 Valuing People: A new strategy for learning disability for the 21st century. NHS Executive, London.

Department of Health 2005 Supporting People with Long-term Conditions: An NHS model to support local innovation and integration. Department of Health, London.

Department of Health 2007 A good practice in learning disability nursing. Department of Health, London.

Department of Health 2007b Progress to transformation: The Big Priorities. Department of Health, London.

Disability Rights Commission 2006 Equal treatment: closing the gap. DRC, London.

Glasby A M 2002 Meeting the needs of people with learning disabilities in acute care. British Journal of Nursing 11(21):1389-1392.

Graham K 2001 Better health care and learning disabilities. Nursing Times 97(8):39-41.

Harries D 1991 A Sense of worth: A report on services for people with learning disabilities and sensory impairments. Committee on the Multi-Handicapped Blind, London.

Hatton C et al 2003 Key Highlights of research evidence on the health of people with learning disabilities. www.valuingpeople.gov.uk/documents/keyhighlights.pdf.

Heyman B, Swain J, Gillman M 2004 Organisational simplification and secondary complexity in health services for adults with learning disabilities. Social Science and Medicine 58:357-367.

Hollins S, Attard M T, von Fraunhofer N, Sedgwick P 1998 Mortality in people with learning disability: risks, causes, and death certification findings in London. Developmental Medicine & Child Neurology 40:50-56.

Howells G 1986 Are the needs of mentally handicapped adults being met? Journal of the Royal College of General Practitioners 36:449-453.

Kerins G, Petrovic K, Gianesini J et al 2004 Physician attitudes and practices on providing care to individuals with intellectual disabilities; an exploratory study. Connecticut Medicine 68:485-490.

Kiernan C 1999 Participation in research by people with learning disabilities: origins and issues. British Journal of Learning Disabilities 27:43-47.

Kuokkanen L, Lerno-Kilpi H 2000 Power and empowerment in nursing: three theoretical approaches. Journal of Advanced Nursing 31(1):235-241.

Lennox N G, Kerr M P 1997 Primary health care and people with an intellectual disability: the evidence base. Journal of Intellectual Disability Research 41(5):365-372.

Lewis R, Dixon J 2004 The future of primary care: meeting the challenges of the new NHS market. Kings Fund, London.

Lindsey M 2002 Comprehensive health care services for people with learning disabilities. Advances in Psychiatric Treatment 8:138-148.

LoBindo-Wood G, Haber J 2002 Nursing research. Methods, critical appraisal and utilization, 5th edn CV Mosby, St Louis.

Martin G 2005 Support for people with learning disabilities: the role of primary care. Primary Care and Community Psychiatry 10(4):133-142.

Martin G H B, Martin D M 2000 A register for patients with learning disabilties in general practice; workload implications of ex-hospital patients. Journal of Learning Disabilities 4:37-48.

McGuigan S M, Hollins S, Attard M 1995 Age specific standardised mortality rates in people with learning disability. Journal of Intellectual Disability Research 39:527-531.

Mencap 2004 Treat me right report: better healthcare for people with learning disability. Mencap, London.

Mencap 2007 Death by indifference report. Mencap, London.

Minihan P M, Dean D H, Lyons C M 1993 Managing the care of patients with mental retardation: A survey of physicians. Mental Retardation 31:239-246.

Office of Public Sector Information 2005 The Mental Capacity Act. OPSI, London.

Office of Public Sector Information 2005 Disability Discrimination Act. OPSI, London.

Powrie E 2003 Primary health care provision for adults with a learning disability. Journal of Advanced Nursing 42(4):413-423.

Prasher V P 1995 Overweight and obesity amongst Down's syndrome adults. Journal of Intellectual Disability Research 39:437-441.

Puri B K, Lekh S K, Langa A et al 1995 Mortality in a hospitalised mentally handicapped population: a 10-year survey. Journal of Intellectual Research 39:442-446.

Rodgers J 1993 Primary health care provision for people with learning disabilities. Health and Social Care 2:11-17.

Roy A, Martin D 1999 A comparative review of primary health with people with learning disabilities. British Journal of Learning Disabilities 25:138-143.

Royal College of Nursing 2006 Meeting the health needs of people with learning disabilities: guidance for nursing staff. RCN, London.

Scottish Executive 2002 Promoting health, supporting inclusion: the national review of the contribution of all nurses and midwives to the care and support of people with learning disabilities.

Primary care and intellectual disability

Sperlinger A 1997 Adults with learning disabilities: a practical approach for health professionals. John Wiley, Chichester.

Thomas K, Velthouse B 1990 Cognitive elements of empowerment: an 'interpretive' model of intrinsic task motivation. Academy of Management Review 15:666-681.

Thornton C, 1999 Effective health care for people with learning disabilities: a formal carers perspective. Journal of Psychiatric Mental Nurse 6:383-390.

Turner N J, Brown A R, Baxter K F 1999 Consent to treatment and the mentally incapacitated adult. Journal of the Royal Society of Medicine 92:290-292.

Walmsely J, Johnson M 2003 Inclusive research with people with learning disabilities: past, present and futures. Jessica Kingsley, London.

Zarb G 1992 On the road to Damascus: first steps towards changing the relations of disability research production. Disability, Handicap and Society 7(2):125-138.

Looks like leisure?

Nick Fripp and Steve Day

Note. Throughout this chapter people are referred to according to their preferred choice of name and with their permission.

'Where you learned how to be not what you are.'

The Eels, Daisies of the Galaxy, 2000

This chapter looks at what leisure is, how people with intellectual disabilities think about and spend their leisure time and how those people who support them attempt to make it happen. The central question is, does this look like leisure? The way leisure is defined is analysed in terms of its relevance to people with intellectual disabilities. This involves discussing the relationship of leisure to work, family and social obligations in the context of the experience of many people with intellectual disabilities. The chapter also explores what services, communities and individuals can contribute in order to support people to be part of the different worlds we all live in. In summary, there are two key objectives to this chapter. The first is to present a Post Modern perspective upon which to understand leisure and people with intellectual disabilities. Secondly the individual narratives and vignettes used will highlight people with intellectual disabilities various perspectives on leisure. This is a short overview of a world that is changing fast.

These discussions take place in today's Post Modern world; a world where some people with intellectual disabilities are discovering their own version of leisure for themselves. While the people who are paid to struggle with funding, inclusion and value-sets do their struggling, people with intellectual disabilities get on with living. This chapter also hears voices from some of those people. It also attempts to weave a set of reflections on leisure in the context of inclusion and people with intellectual disabilities. We consider the traditional response from 'service-land' (the local government reality of assessments, Working Party responses and off the shelf services) to the challenge of enabling specific, individual people to go out into their communities and 'get a life'.

POSTMODERNITY

What is meant by the term 'Post Modern'? In trying to define Post-Modernity, Thomas Docherty talks about 'an ambiguity' surrounding the phrase. He traces its history back to Arnold Toynbee's writing in 1939 (*A Study In History*) and then on through a trail of academic study, from the Enlightenment to

LIVERPOOL JOHN MOORES UNIVERSITY
LEARNING SERVICES

Marxism, before arriving at the statement, 'on the other hand it is simply a desire, a mood which looks to the future to redeem the present' (Docherty 1993:2). Our PostModern world is ambiguous; the old certainties have disappeared leaving us with a desire for definition in a society where everything appears to constantly seek redefinition in order to suit the presenting circumstance.

In attempting to put a time-frame on what we mean by 'a Post Modern world' we are writing about the period, after modernity, after air flight, after abstraction, after the absence of innocence and the war to end all wars. Modernity took hold in terms of a belief in the early 20th century; technological and scientific progress would lead to a future where leisure time was something more and more people would have more and more of. The beginning of PostModernity can be traced to the early 1940s; the pleasures of plenty which had arrived with modernity began to look distinctly uncomfortable with Europe under occupation. As a new global realignment emerged so too did the values by which people defined themselves. Post-Modernity does not come with one clear definition, however it has its roots in the desire to throw out the old certainties of elite empires in favour of a rough and ready pragmatism. The potential was there for leisure, like everything else, to be whatever you wanted it to be.

In Best & Kellner's critique of Post-Modernism they write of its 'limitations and distortions' (Best & Kellner 1991:275). Are not limitations and distortions increasingly recognisable everywhere? Today such a question is almost commonplace. And so we write about personal leisure alongside the personal suicide bomber's explosion. This chapter's exploration of leisure and people with intellectual disabilities refuses to accept the lazy rhetoric that all people with intellectual disabilities want to work, become tenants and be included in their community. People with intellectual disabilities live in the same world characterised by Beavis and Butt-Head. A world where young people are seen by Best & Kellner (1998:74) as, 'a large teenage underclass that is undereducated; that comes from broken homes; that is angry, resentful, and potentially violent and that has nothing to do but to engage in social mayhem'.

People with intellectual disabilities are included in this world of distortions and leisure is one of its limitations. The exploration of issues for people with intellectual disabilities can be liberated when seen through a Post Modern filter. The world of modernity was a world which embraced eugenics; Post-Modernity offers us all a second chance. While Post-Modernism may be ambiguous and to some extent indefinable it offers the opportunity for new and inclusive paradigms to emerge. Through this fog of ambiguity we begin to discover a platform upon which to understand the leisure issues faced by people with intellectual disabilities.

WHAT IS LEISURE?

Bull et al (2003) note that leisure is becoming increasingly important in the lives of many people because of decreasing time spent at work and increasing disposable income. They identify four major approaches to defining leisure:

- *Time-based approaches* see leisure as the time not spent at work or meeting basic needs for survival (sleep, eating etc.).
- *Activity-based approaches* define leisure in terms of activities that are not daily necessities or obligations in the context of family, social or employment responsibilities.
- *Attitude-based approaches* are informed by the varying definitions of individuals about what leisure is. This approach sees leisure in terms of how a person perceives what is going on rather than in terms of location, time or activity.
- *Quality-based approaches* attribute affective characteristics to activities. An activity could be described as leisure if it is associated with freedom, physical activity, pleasure, relaxation or creativity.

In terms of the time- or activity-based definitions, many people with intellectual disabilities would be leisure participants for most of their lives. The range of opportunities for inclusion in terms of employment, ' . . . less than 10% [of people with intellectual disabilities] nationally are in work . . .' (Department of Health 2001), and the exercising of responsibility in the context of family and leadership roles are often very limited. What may be seen as leisure activities defined in terms of the quality of the experience often take place in the context of services that actually isolate people and provide none of the counterpoints to activities which help to define leisure as something that is personal, choice based and free of externally imposed obligations. Some of these services were described in Valuing People:

> 'Day services frequently fail to provide sufficiently flexible and individual support. Some large day centres offer little more than warehousing and do not help people with learning disabilities undertake a wider range of individually tailored activities. Social isolation remains a problem for too many people with learning disabilities. A recent study found that only 30% had a friend who was not either learning disabled, or part of their family or paid to care for them.'
>
> Department of Health 2001

Mike used to go to a traditional day centre; however, he decided that it no longer offered him the kind of experiences he was interested in. Mike does not break down his time in a way that separates leisure from the rest of his life. He is an adult with intellectual disabilities not engaging in activities that are 'provided' by statutory agencies. The opportunity arose to interview Mike about leisure. These are the notes recorded directly after that meeting:

I asked him whether the weekend had gone well. However, he was not in a position to comment. Mike had no idea where he was in the weekly cycle. Saturday and Sunday had passed him by without declaring their identity. This state of affairs was not because his 'intellectual disability' had divorced him from the days of the week, he just had a different attitude to time and space, or at least how I label each twenty-four hours as they continually come round. 'It's all the same to me, I'm too busy.' For months now Mike has been working on his car. He will never drive it. Mike's

9

hatchback has a much more interesting function. 'I call it Brian because it isn't going anywhere. I'm rebuilding the car as a sculpture.' The vehicle is 'parked' on the drive, one wheel without a tyre, the whole thing permanently propped up on bricks. Mike has painted the dented bodywork a variety of different colours. The interior looks like a gap in a mouth where a tooth's been pulled. 'No, I am not in any hurry. My attitude is, this is what I do. And I do it every day.' He did not actually use the word, but Mike defines himself by his car. And yes, he did use the word 'attitude', which caused me to make some notes. I wrote on the back of a petrol receipt, 'Too busy but not in any hurry.'

There is a recurring theme in literature exploring leisure and relationships for people with intellectual disabilities that suggests that many people with intellectual disabilities have a solitary and lonely experience of time passing without purpose (Cheseldine & Jeffree 1981, McConkey et al 1981 cited by Cavet 1995, Oswin 1971). Bayley (1997:32) found during his study of friendship that:

> 'An overwhelming impression from the project was that many people with learning difficulties find time a burden not a gift – whether it was Arthur Needles watching television all day in the sitting room at his parent's house, Christopher Johnson lying on the sitting room floor playing with his sock, or Philip Brindley and Jason Havering in their pleasant house watching television programmes that did not interest them . . .'

This sense of time ebbing away with nothing to show for it is by no means a concept that is confined to the literature of the late 20th century as the following example from 2007 shows:

A day service provider recently suggested that if a certain person was not able to attend the day centre they ran they would spend all day 'staring at the walls'. I talked to the manager of the service where this person lived about this statement – 'tell me it ain't so!!' In many ways it was so. The care manager had suggested a solution that involves travelling to a day centre two days per week which involves a 1.5 hour round trip. The question becomes even more exasperating – is this person really spending their life staring at the walls? Is the only salvation one which involves staff spending 3 hours per day transporting the person to and from a day centre that is miles away? Even if it is what happens on the other 5 days per week?

A new solution was proposed – a person-centred plan will be developed that will explore who the person is, how they want to enjoy their time and how people can support this person on the basis of what is learned.

Staggeringly we must still assume nothing in terms of whether people are being supported to get a life. Whoever you are, do not accept that staring at walls is good enough.

Wolfensberger's (1991) concept of the wound of 'life wasting' characterises some the particularly negative imagery around time use. The story above shows that such life wasting has not gone away.

EACH PERSON DEFINES THEIR OWN VERSION OF LEISURE

The following script is presented as a contrast to the imagery of tragedy and low expectations and stigma which is, of course, in the eye of the beholder. Many people today disregard the polarisation of work and leisure; for people with intellectual disabilities the two concepts merge, often because their lifestyles are not compartmentalised into these two definite activities. These themes come to light in this discussion between members of North Somerset People First, a self-advocacy group for people with intellectual disabilities. In this conversation individual versions of leisure can appear to be almost contradictory.

North Somerset People First speak about leisure

Phillip risks the first definition, 'I guess, mmm, leisure is what you do in your own time.' Silence. We all look at each other around the table. It is a good place to start but no one is really sure whether this is quite sufficient.

I make the obvious reply, 'Okay, if there is a period which is 'your own time' what is happening in this 'other time'?'

Mark Smith, the current Chairperson of North Somerset People First, provides the answer, 'Well, that's when you are working or at college, stuff like that . . .'

'Or at the day centre,' says Nicola Ann Counsell.

'So, you don't see going to the day centre as leisure time?'

She chuckles, 'Not at all, the day centre can be hard work. I go because that is what I do but it's not like . . . not like a holiday!'

Martin has been giving the matter some thought, 'Leisure is about choosing what you want to do, having some control of what you do and what order you do it.'

'Socialising comes into it,' says Phillip, 'People socialise at work, get along with each other, there's a difference.'

I try to get some clarity on the issue, 'How about this People First meeting, is this leisure?'

'No way,' says Mark, 'It can be a laugh but . . .'

'We have to do business, it can be fun but we are here to make decisions.' Martin brings the conversation back to his original point, 'In your leisure time, it's about choice, you can choose what you do.'

This prompts the group into thinking about what they like doing in their 'leisure time'.

Phillip: 'Exercising, watching horse racing and Formula One; The Simpson's.'

Nicola: 'I enjoy writing stories.'

Mark: 'Going out, just going out.'

Martin: 'When I was working at B&Q, I sometimes felt trapped by the customers. I was glad to get home, just to have some space to myself.'

Opposite Martin, on the other side of the table Katherine Sawyer has been listening to the conversation. She is particularly interested in what Martin is talking about. When I ask Katherine what she does in her leisure time she replies, 'Working at McDonalds.'

I make the mistake of trying to correct Katherine's answer. 'Isn't that your work time?'

Continued

Looks like leisure?

North Somerset People First speak about leisure—cont'd

'No, I really enjoy my job. I do three hours at their busiest time. I get to meet lots of different people. It feels enjoyable. When I get home I am worn out, but when I am at work I am having a good time.'

'She's achieving something,' says Mark.

'I am,' agrees Katherine, 'I really am.'

'This is interesting,' I am muttering and writing words down quickly in a note-book, underlining and drawing arrows. 'It feels as if we are turning leisure and work upside down.'

Martin is sat next to me and is looking at my page of scribbles. He reminds me again, 'We choose how we see things.'

At the other end of the table is Ian Timothy-Brooks. Until now Ian has not said anything although he has been very attentive to what everyone else has been saying. Ian now tells the group what he likes doing in his 'leisure time'. 'I like it when my Dad visits me at the weekend. We go out into town. Have a drink at the Conservative Club. Sometimes buy things. We meet my brother and his girlfriend. Have a meal. I used to like going to the beach. The open air, watching the tide, I used to feel free on the beach.'

'This sounds good.' I then ask a question, 'What is it that you particularly like, Ian? Is it about seeing your Dad or is it about the things you do with him?'

'I like seeing Dad that's important, but I enjoy just being able to go out like everybody else.'

'Would you like to go out more?'

'Yes, of course.'

We finish off the conversation with a wish list. If the people in the group all had lots of money, millions of pounds to spend, and could do anything they liked what would they do.

Nicola: 'Go back to Austria, I would like to try hang-gliding.'

Phillip: 'I'd like to do lots of things to my house.'

Katherine: 'Watch Liverpool, watch them play in Liverpool.'

Mark: 'Visit Croatia for a holiday, I've been before.'

Ian: 'Buy a boat; a proper boat, a cruiser, a large boat.'

Martin: 'I'd choose something special. I need to really think about it.'

THE ANALYSIS

Mark, Nicola, Phillip, Martin, Katherine and Ian discuss leisure like it is the most normal thing in the world. No one requires an explanation or a definition of the word 'leisure'. Each of them has their own individual ideas about what the meaning might be of leisure in the UK towards the end of the first decade of the 21st century. For the citizens of a Post Modern western society, fragmented by its leaders' inability to focus on building stability, leisure can be taken for granted even if it looks different to different people. Even if leisure is working in McDonald's or watching the Simpson's; people with intellectual disabilities, like other social groups, are having to take matters into their own hands – or at least their own thinking. While professionals are paid to assess and report in order to find funding for inclusion while talking concepts of person centredness, people with intellectual disabilities get on with their lives in ways that make sense to them.

Absurdity is a mirage from a bygone age. When Katherine Sawyer talks of finding leisure in her work at McDonald's she is not being deliberately obtuse or consciously wishing to redefine the difference between perception and reality. She is merely exercising her desire to live her life in a way that feels comfortable to her. Like the rest of her colleagues in North Somerset People First, Katherine Sawyer asserts her individuality. Work equals leisure if you want it too. In an uncertain world where meaning is either intensely personal or globally political, where peace-keeping and war-making are often indistinguishable and organic is panic, terms such as leisure are merely relative. Depending on who you are and where you are and what you believe, leisure is going to feel very different.

TAKING A YEAR OFF

In the course of exploring the concept of leisure Nash (1953, cited by Hogg & Cavet 1995) asked people what they would do with a year off. He recorded some of the things people told him, 'Here they are writing poetry, building a cabin, making a piece of poetry, singing a song, playing the ukulele, painting a picture, sailing a boat . . . They go to the ends of the earth to see canyons, climb mountains, chase caribou, follow migratory birds, dig dinosaur eggs in the Gobi desert . . .' In considering this question for people with intellectual disabilities it is worth asking, a year off from what?

Hogg & Cavet (1995) explore definitions of leisure for people with profound intellectual and multiple disabilities and seek definitions that are based on choice and the non-obligatory nature of leisure instead of definitions of leisure in terms of time not spent at work. Hogg & Cavet (1995) review Nash's 1957 hierarchical scheme of leisure participation which runs through a numerical scale from sub zero, which represents acts against society, to creative participation (Table 9.1).

Hogg & Cavet (1995) develop a non-hierarchical model, retaining the four above zero activity areas but moving away from attaching relative value or status to any of them.

Hogg's ecology of leisure for people includes carers; for many people with intellectual disabilities the mapping of relationships will mean that leisure today will need to be considered in the context of a world that has been created for people rather than chosen by them. Like a well-drawn PATH (Planning Alternative Tomorrows with Hope), processing the vision becomes the starting point toward a positive outcome. Possible goals are the steps taken on the journey. PATH is just one of several different models of approaching Person

Looks like leisure?

Table 9.1	Nash's 1957 hierarchical scheme of leisure participation
Sub zero	Acts against society
Zero	Injury or detriment to self or others [life wasting perhaps?]
One	Killing time, amusement, entertainment and escape from monotony
Two	Emotional participation (watching, appreciating)
Three	Active participation (playing the part, copying the model)
Four	Creative participation (the maker of the model, composer, artist, inventor)

Centred Planning. Its key value is that it allows someone to pictorially chart the journey they need to take in order to reach what they want to achieve. In this context simply wishing away the service created environment that some people live in is to ignore people's reality. Dowson (1998:20) reviews the role of leisure in day centres and concludes, '. . . days spent in leisure pursuits do not represent 'living like other people' – especially when low income is a bar to many activities.' Planning with friends and family a pictorial route to inclusion and the identification of personal goals are the practical first steps away from being dominated by 'services'.

SO WHAT CAN AND IS BEING DONE ABOUT LEISURE AND INCLUSION?

Most importantly people with intellectual disabilities are getting a life, not being supported or being given permission to have one. The phrase 'getting a life' might seem merely colloquial, but it represents the idea of personal discovery, finding that particular set of leisure pleasures which resonate for you. Fortunately people's lives have the capacity to take on a shape that is uniquely personal.

Case study 9.1   Julia's story

I enjoy doing lots of things; cooking – spaghetti bolognaise is my favourite, shopping – I like buying CDs and DVDs. I often choose the CDs we play in the car. I like Tina Turner because she has got a big voice. I also buy lots of DVDs. I like watching horror films, Nightmare On Elm Street is the best because I like all the scary bits when people get killed by 'Freddy'. It's like having a bad nightmare but I know it's not real. I enjoy it, the scarier the better.

Two decades ago Julia's liking for horror films may have been discouraged. Wolfensberger's Conservatism Corollary (Wolfensberger & Thomas, 1983) can be interpreted to suggest that human service workers overcompensate to reduce or minimise any 'devaluing characteristics' or features of a person's appearance or behaviour. In this context Julia may perhaps have been encouraged to follow a more conservative leisure choice such as the teachings of Dot Cotton in East Enders or the world view of Ken Barlow in Coronation Street.

Julia is getting on with her life. So what is the role of support providers? Firstly it is important to ensure that leisure does not become institutionalised. Whatever the definition leisure should not and cannot be the product of an institution or agency. It should always be defined by the individual concerned. Buttimer & Tierney (2005:36) warn of 'A tendency for everyday activities to become scrutinized and therefore become medicalised, e.g. art becomes art therapy, gardening becomes horticultural therapy, music becomes music therapy'. While the business of manipulating environments for children to develop the skills to participate in leisure activities is an appropriate feature of the school curriculum (Yalon-Chamovitz et al 2006) it is important that we do not continue to imagine that adults need to continue to learn until they 'fit in'.

The staring at the walls story above illustrates a shift from doing for and deciding for towards person centred thinking and the simple business of finding out what people want before we plan their lives.

ASSET-BASED COMMUNITY DEVELOPMENT

In seeking to answer the challenge of how can we find ways for people to share their gifts, Asset-Based Community Development (ABCD) offers one way forward. ABCD draws on the thinking of John McKnight for example in Kretzmann et al (2005) and Green et al (2006). It does not suggest that organisations, associations or agencies do it for people but that they use their assets to amplify assets that are already in the community. As in Person Centred Planning, the ABCD approach places value on the individual and the fragmented world in which they live. Those fragments can be turned into potential assets and used to chart a personal contribution within community involvement. Carl Poll (2003) reflected on key lessons learned during his 15 years working with Key Ring. 'Firstly that people with learning disabilities (all of them) have gifts, second that communities (all of them) have good things going on in them. I'm still learning a third which is about how to link the two.'

The following story records the experience of two people and seems to be a great example of what ABCD can achieve. Ian Callen co-ordinates an educational project in a public park and Jason Evans is a student on a horticultural course at the project.

Looks like leisure?

Ian said:
It started how these things often do – just an idea. 3 months before Christmas we thought let's have a carol service. Tracy [Ian's boss] suggested that we hold it in the swimming pool garden (which is a community space in the park). I put the word out and people started getting in touch, 'I can bring candles!', 'I can bring lanterns!', 'I can tell stories!', 'I am in a singing chorus!', 'I want to sing a solo'. There was lots of interest.

Jason said:
When the solo started I went down the steps. I was a bit shaken up. I was nervous to sing the song. Then I relaxed and just sang the whole song through. It is good skills to sing the song. I picked Driving Home for Christmas because it gives you good memories – people seeing families and stuff. I was so happy and glad I was crying during the song. There were lots of people behind me in the chorus, I was comfortable with that. At home I have a picture of me singing the song [in News 2 U, a Brandon Trust Newsletter]. It said Jason Evans was fantastic.

The recipe for success was in Ian's words having an enthusiastic line manager who lets you go – lets you follow ideas up. The location is really important. The project is based in a public park which is a focal point for the community. There is also a local group of people who love the park called the Eastville Park Action Group. Finally it is important to have a passion for community and what it means – not just being in it but being part of it.

This is a great example of an agency facilitating community building. The asset of the organisation was presence, time to organise and the development skills and passion for community action of the staff. Community members' gifts were critical to the success of the event and one of those people, Jason, got to enjoy his leisure time doing what he likes to do.

There are other positive examples of initiatives that start from the position of equal access to leisure and supporting mainstream agencies to learn how to welcome community members with intellectual disabilities. Easton (2002) describes the Inclusive Fitness Initiative which is designed to support leisure centres to adopt and put into practice policies that will enable all disabled people to be included. The initiative offers training to staff working in leisure centres and guidance on marketing the benefits and availability of fitness to disabled people. The sophisticated, evidence based approach aims to ensure that mainstream amenities can accommodate the support requirements of disabled people. This is achieved through both changing the equipment and physical environment and also the culture change that is needed to welcome disabled people, 'Negative attitudes and culture are perhaps the greatest bars to participation in this type of leisure pursuit' (Easton 2003:19). Livesey (2003) records the experiences of the Bringing Leisure Alive project in Glasgow. Following consultation with people with intellectual disabilities, families and carers access to leisure was identified as a priority. Training is offered to staff working with people with intellectual disabilities and the aim of the project is to work towards a vision that foresees, 'When they have time to spare, people with intellectual difficulties will be able to access leisure in the same way as other citizens, having open and accessible facilities, being treated with dignity and respect and being included.'

A further positive example of exploring life outside a segregated setting as part of day service modernisation is presented by Nielsen & Porter (2002) who recorded the experience of a group of people with intellectual disabilities who tried activities in their local community as an alternative to their day centre.

Alongside improving access to mainstream facilities there continues to be a range of specialist arrangements for people with intellectual disabilities – Snoezelen, Gateway Clubs, Befriending Schemes, Community Use sessions in Day Service Programmes. Hogg & Cavet (1995) provide a thorough review of research, approaches and practice in this respect. They note that people with profound intellectual disabilities and multiple impairments are often not addressed by inclusion initiatives. It is not, of course, the case that this group of people need to be served in segregated settings despite the fact that one of the attitudinal barriers identified in Making it Happen (Mencap 1997:16) seems all too familiar, ' . . . severely disabled people are best left to the professionals because they know what they are doing'. Making it Happen not only identifies barriers but suggests ways to overcome them. It makes practical recommendations for action for inclusion including a central information resource, national standards for accessibility and calls for leisure organisations to consider and address the requirements and interests of people with profound intellectual disabilities.

People with intellectual disabilities are not just waiting for leisure providers to get it right they are increasingly taking on the job of sorting out their own events. There are a growing number of club nights run by and for people with intellectual disabilities.

'I felt nervous when I got on stage but then I thought, 'sod this, I'm raring to go' and just got on with it.'

'I like the Halloween gig because I'm part of the Wild Bunch organising team – emailing people, getting flyers out on time, making it happen. Everyone makes an effort which makes it the biggest event of the year – 250 people come! There's a blinding atmosphere in the DJ area and the dance floor is full of people with fancy dress costumes. It's a bit frightening and scary but everyone's having a good time and everything is running smoothly.'

Community Living 2003, issues 16(4) and 17(1)

Leisure is what we make it. Leisure goes on inside our heads. Leisure is when we stretch our minds out of the tight corners and let ourselves go. Whether this happens during some high performance sport, or couched in front of the telly or singing in the park, or even crying in the park, in essence it is all part of the same process. At the beginning of this chapter it is suggested that a Post Modern perspective involves unravelling our old certainties about what constitutes leisure. Having done this the premise takes on a new clarity, leisure is wherever we personally find it. Examine leisure for what it is but do not feel constrained by what other people, including authors of chapters on Leisure, label it as. Many people with intellectual difficulties experience the pleasure principle outside of the worklife balance and in doing so they provide a model for the rest of us.

REFERENCES

Bayley M 1997 What price friendship? Encouraging the relationships of people with learning difficulties. Hexagon, Minehead.

Best S, Kellner D 1991 Postmodern theory: critical interrogations. Macmillan, London.

Best S, Kellner D 1998 Beavis and Butt-Head: no future for postmodern youth. In: Epstein J S (ed) Youth culture in a postmodern world. Blackwell, Oxford.

Bull C, Hoose J, Weed M 2003 An introduction to leisure studies. Pearson Education, Harlow.

Buttimer J, Tierney E 2005 Patterns of leisure participation among adolescents with a mild learning disability. Journal of Intellectual Disabilities Research 9(1):25-42.

Cavet J 1995 Sources of information about the leisure of people with profound and multiple disabilities. In: Hogg J, Cavet J (eds) Making leisure provision for people with profound learning and multiple disabilities. Chapman and Hall, London.

Cheseldine S, Jeffree D 1981 Mentally handicapped adolescents: their use of leisure. Journal of Mental Deficiency Research 25:49-59.

Department of Health 2001 Valuing People: a new strategy for learning disability for the 21st century. Department of Health, London.

Docherty T (ed) 1993 Postmodernism: a reader. Columbia University Press, New York.

Dowson S 1998 Certainties without centres? A discussion paper on day services for people who have learning difficulties. Values Into Action, London.

Easton C 2002 Fitness for all. Living Well 2(2):17-22.

Green M, Moore H, O'Brien J 2006 When people care enough to act. Inclusion Press, Toronto.

Hogg J, Cavet J (eds) 1995 Making leisure provision for people with profound learning and multiple disabilities. Chapman & Hall.

Kretzmann J, McKnight J, Dobrowolski S, Puntenney D 2005 Discovering community power: a guide to mobilizing local assets and your organization's capacity. ABCD Institute, Evanston.

Livesey C 2003 Bringing Leisure Alive: improving access to leisure for people with learning difficulties in Glasgow. Living Well 3(2):27-30.

Nielsen P, Porter S 2002 Without walls – not without opportunities. Living Well 2(4):14-18.

Oswin M 1971 The empty hours. Penguin, London.

Poll C 2003 People with learning difficulties and community – two things worth knowing. Living Well 3(3):4-9.

Wolfensberger W 1991 A brief introduction to social role valorization as a high-order concept for structuring human services. Center for Human Policy, Syracuse.

Wolfensberger W, Thomas S 1983 PASSING (Program Analysis of Service Systems' Implementation of Normalization Goals): Normalization criteria and ratings manual. National Institute on Mental Retardation, Toronto.

Yalon-Chamovitz S, Mano T, Jarus T, Weinblatt N 2006 Leisure activities during school breaks among children with learning disabilities: preferences vs. performance. British Journal of Learning Disabilities 34(1):42-49.

Getting into employment

Sarah Maguire

10

INTRODUCTION

The 'Monday morning blues' is a unifying factor for more than 23 million adults in the United Kingdom (UK) as they begin their working week. Despite our propensity to 'moan' about work, I am sure most of us would not readily give up the rewards that we derive from it. Work is an integral part of most of our adult lives. It brings with it not just financial rewards but the benefits of helping us feel good about ourselves. Most of us increase our social networks through work and many go on to meet our future partners (Department of Work and Pensions 2002:v).

However, work is still not an integral part of the lives of people with intellectual disabilities in the UK. It is over 30 years since the King's Fund published 'An Ordinary Working Life' (1984) and began to challenge assumptions about people with intellectual disabilities' rights to work. The first National Survey of Adults with Learning Difficulties (Emerson et al 2005:47–48) showed that, of the 2898 people interviewed, only one in six (17%) had a paid job, compared to 67% of men and 53% of women of working age without intellectual disabilities in the UK.

The 'Working Lives' study into the role of day centres in supporting people with intellectual disabilities into employment (Beyer et al 2004, cited in Department for Work and Pensions 2006:9) found that most people they interviewed wanted to work, even if they are not working at present, and they mainly wanted paid work.

This poses a question about the number and range of initiatives designed to specifically increase employment opportunities for people with intellectual disabilities. This section will offer a brief overview of the legislation that relates to employment opportunities for people with intellectual disabilities. In 2001 the Department of Health's 'Valuing People' strategy made clear its objective to:

> 'enable more people with learning disabilities to participate in all forms of employment wherever possible in paid work, and to make a valued contribution to the world of work'.
>
> Department of Health 2001:8

The strategy outlined its intention to introduce a range of new initiatives to remove some of the barriers to employment for people with disabilities e.g., Workstep programmes aimed at providing individually tailored packages of support for people with disabilities, Job Brokers, New Deal for Disabled People, better links between Department of Health and Department for Education and Employment. Two years later in 2003, the Department for Work and Pensions published its proposals for new 'Pathways to Work'. The document acknowledged that, despite making some headway, still more needed to be done to support people with disabilities to share in the employment successes brought about by welfare reform (Department for Work and Pensions 2003:6). We have also seen changes in the law in relation to employment with the Disability Discrimination Act 1995 and 2005 which shifted the burden of proof in discrimination cases from the disabled person to the employer (Disability Rights Commission 2005). Finally, in 2005 'Improving the Life Chances of Disabled People' was published, reinforcing this Government's inclusion agenda by stating that, by 2025, disabled people in Britain would be respected and included as equal members of society (Prime Minister's Strategy Unit 2005:3). It could be argued that this leaves us 18 years to achieve what we have been struggling with for the past 30 years.

Despite task force after task force, initiative after initiative, policy after policy, people with intellectual disabilities are still finding it hard to get a job. Ian Davies and Karen Spencer from Central England People First Research were part of the team of researchers working on the first National Survey of Adults with Learning Difficulties in England (2003/4). They were not surprised by the results of the Survey and said that, in their experience, people received poor support and information (Emerson et al 2005:47). This appears to be borne out in the Survey results, with only 9% of people having heard about specific programmes like Workstep, aimed at getting disabled people who are long term unemployed into work (Emerson et al 2005:114). Also, 25% of people surveyed said they would seek help and advice on looking for work from their parents and support staff, compared with 5% who would use the Job Centre/Connexions service (Emerson et al 2005:115).

This raises an important issue about inclusion – do 'specialist' initiatives and projects keep people with intellectual disabilities segregated from mainstream employment opportunities and create more challenges than they solve? Or is it the way specialist services are structured, and who they align themselves with that has the potential to offer more opportunities for employment?

The employment challenges for people with intellectual disabilities are numerous and well documented in the recent report to the 'Learning Disability Task' force by the Working Group on Learning Disabilities and Employment (Department for Work and Pensions 2006). A common thread through this report is the connection between employment and the wider community. Although not an answer in itself, maybe closer links with local communities could create more employment opportunities for people with intellectual disabilities.

This chapter aims to examine some of the barriers to employment for people with intellectual disabilities. The chapter will look at:

- Employment and its effect on self esteem
- Employers' perceptions of people with disabilities
- The perceptions of individuals with intellectual disabilities about employment

- The range of government initiatives to increase employment opportunities for people with intellectual disabilities
- Building inclusive communities and community partnerships to increase employment opportunities for people with intellectual disabilities

Most importantly, this chapter will shares stories and views of people with intellectual disabilities about their own personal experience of the world of employment.

BUILDING INCLUSIVE COMMUNITIES

There are still many obstacles which prevent people with intellectual disabilities from playing a full and active part in their communities and at work. People have mostly been separated from their communities by long-stay hospitals, segregated schooling and continue to experience separate activities. This has led to, and continues to engender, a lack of understanding about the contribution that people can make, and about their capabilities and aspirations. Against this background, it is important that employment is not viewed as a means to an end in itself, but a vital factor in building a healthy community. If people with intellectual disabilities are excluded from opportunities to work, they cannot fully participate in society. Supporting people into work can contribute significantly to fostering social cohesion and involving people in their communities.

Micro Enterprises is an idea that started in the USA and has been championed by the National Development Team for People with Learning Disabilities (NDT) for the past 3–4 years. I went along to one of their seminars 3 years ago to listen to the architects of this new approach, Doreen Rosimos and Darcy Smith, and was immediately struck by the link between meaningful, flexible employment for people with intellectual disabilities and their connections to their local community (National Development Team 2007).

A micro enterprise is a small business venture. They are concerned about getting a job, not for the sake of it, but to help people become richer, have more purposeful lives and provide new connections with their local community. A successful micro enterprise is one where the person is at the centre and we consider their interests in relation to their community. The aim of the micro enterprise is to make money by seeking out ordinary community opportunities. The business is usually owned by one person and only requires a small amount of capital to set up – usually £200–£300.

This approach has proved successful for many individuals in the USA and UK alike and was reflected in the views of people interviewed as part of the Working Lives study (Beyer et al 2004). This study highlighted that:

'Whilst earning money was a major motivation they also clearly stated the importance of having a job in supporting social contact and making a contribution to their community.'

Many people with intellectual disabilities have begun to think about setting up their own businesses. Bev has given her permission to share the story of her micro enterprise.

Case study 10.1 'A business of my own' – Bev's story

Bev moved out of Fieldhead Hospital in Wakefield to her own home in 2004. In the three years she has lived in her new home she has developed a great deal of independence and control of her life. Most people, Bev included, never believed she would be able to live on her own. They felt she would be unable to cope, that her 'behaviours' would lead to all sorts of trouble with her neighbours and get in the way of making friends and getting a job.

Bev has proved everyone wrong and is very proud of her achievements. However not all of her life is as she would like it. Because Bev lives on her own, she often faces difficulties paying her bills. Bev is often lonely and gets bored being at home alone for long periods of time. She has worked really hard to shake off the label of having 'challenging behaviour' and is able to cope with her emotions and stop them interfering with her life. However, Bev's emotions have got in the way of her seeking a traditional '9 to 5' job.

Bev and her support team had spent a lot of time thinking about ways of solving this problem when they heard about some funding available to set up a micro enterprise. The funding was from Bev's support provider, who was keen to support employment initiatives. Bev put in a proposal to set up a card making business. This was something she was already interested in and had already sold some of her early work to friends. Bev found people liked her designs and she sold more to staff in her support provider's local office.

When the micro enterprise idea came along Bev jumped at the idea. She used the money to pay for more materials and to attend a craft class at her local college to learn new techniques. Through her previous sales and a new network she established at college, Bev has found a whole new market for her business. She is hoping to run a craft stall in her local market later this year.

Bev had never been in a position to go into paid employment, but since leaving hospital and developing her card making business, she now says she wants to look at other employment opportunities. Bev says that setting up her micro enterprise has helped her fill her time; make new friends and connections with her neighbours and people around where she lives; helped her save for things she struggled to afford like a holiday; made her feel good about herself because people liked her designs and have paid her to do more. Bev has a new-found confidence in herself and her future in paid employment.

A lack of confidence can be a major factor in limiting employment opportunities for people with intellectual disabilities.

So much effort has been made by Learning Disability Partnership Boards to write employment strategies (Grove & Mackintosh 2005). So many evaluations have taken place on the role day services play in supporting employment (Beyer et al 2004). Has all this effort been rewarded by seeing growing numbers of people with intellectual disabilities in employment? If we compare the cost of an average day centre placement (£1000s) with the cost of Bev's micro enterprise grant (£200), one has to ask if her self determined approach has been more effective and efficient in terms of cost.

We already know from the survey carried out by Central England People First and Eric Emerson (2005), that people with intellectual disabilities are more likely to ask their family, friends or support staff how to get a job than seek advice from employment specialist like the Job Centre or Connexions. If this is the case, has the extensive raft of initiatives, services and policy documents made employment less accessible to people with intellectual disabilities and their supporters?

The findings of the Working Group on Learning Disabilities and Employment (2006) suggest that all such policies have not been futile. They welcomed the proactive attitude local authorities and voluntary organisations have taken to employment and praised local initiatives as part of the day centre modernisation programme and 'Valuing People' agenda (Department for Work and Pensions 2006:280). However, they recognised the scarce resources at the disposal of most local authorities. The report goes on to stress that people need proper resources to be delivered to where they live – their local community. As such the Government is now considering transferring the responsibility for employment for people with intellectual disabilities from the local authorities to the Department for Work and Pensions (Department for Work and Pensions 2006:29). If intellectual disability services continue to look to their local Partnership Boards or commissioners for help with employment, there is a danger that intellectual disability services do not become fully engaged with the opportunities the wider community can offer.

This idea is being pioneered by the 'In Control' programme in its community building programme (Kennedy et al 2004:1). The 'In Control' programme talks about the importance of active citizenship and the concerns expressed by many people with intellectual disabilities about their exclusion from this process. 'In Control' is encouraging local authorities to sign up to their 'Small Sparks' community building programme (Poll 2005). This is a simple idea where an organisation like a local authority offers a small grant of up to £250 to individuals who have an idea for a project to improve their local community. People have to match the £250. They can do this in funding through a donation from a local business, in materials, labour or time. In 2005, some of the Small Sparks projects included a sponsored cycle ride, sharing craft ideas, making a sensory garden, ladies' football, skittle competition, under-5s sports day, musical evening and a 'get to know your neighbour' event. While there is increasing acknowledgement that people with intellectual disabilities are able to work, the majority of people with intellectual disabilities, and particularly people with severe intellectual disabilities, continue to rely on day centres, from where there is often limited, if any, opportunity to move to employment.

A substantial majority of people spend a lot of time in volunteer placements that, like their day centre, do not lead on to jobs. If this is the case, do projects like Small Sparks offer a different type of voluntary work experience that places the individual at the heart of their community? They also have the potential to lead on to other work opportunities as in Bev's case.

With community cohesion high on the agenda, it is important that people with intellectual disabilities are kept in the loop. The more people with intellectual disabilities are supported to participate in their communities, the more visible their needs and contributions will be and the need to consider them in any plans. In this context there is a job to be done to increase awareness and understanding of the successes of paid employment, that includes publicising work to employers, training projects, care managers and support services and to the wider community (Beyer et al 2004). It is exactly this approach that Toucan Employment have been taking for the past 18 years.

BUILDING COMMUNITY PARTNERSHIPS

Toucan Employment is a small specialist employment agency based in the London borough of Southwark. Established in 1989, it has been quietly supporting hundreds of people with intellectual disabilities to take up paid jobs with a diverse range of employers, including the Ministry of Defence, House of Commons, Royal Festival Hall, Urban Outfitters and B&Q.

Toucan's Managing Director, Ray Whitikker, is clear that to help people get local jobs, it is essential to both understand, and be a part of, that local community. Ray believes that employment for people with intellectual disabilities is as much about changing attitudes as it is about finding an actual job. It is important to challenge negative, stereotypic perceptions about people with intellectual disabilities. In 2004, the Disability Rights Commission carried out some research on attitudes towards employing people with disabilities, involving 1000 small businesses. They found that when 41% of the employers surveyed heard the word ' disabled', they immediately thought of a person who used a wheelchair. The reality is that 1 in 3 of the 10 million disabled people in Britain uses a wheelchair.

Toucan feel they have an important role to play in challenging these attitudes. They have opened a successful café in the heart of their local community. Café Van Gogh is different from other 'training' café's for people with intellectual disabilities as it was set up to be a commercially viable venture that offered employment opportunities to all local people. There is nothing 'specialist' about Café Van Gogh. In a very ordinary way, with no fanfares or banners, the café is challenging and changing the attitudes of the community and its potential employers towards people with intellectual disabilities. But it is not just the attitudes of the community and employers that Toucan have to tackle. Mark has worked at the café for some months, but has found getting a job really hard:

'I did do an interview; I think it was Tesco. It wasn't very good, I'm afraid. I never really wanted to go in the first place. I felt a bit low down.'

It is common for people with intellectual disabilities themselves to believe that they will not be able to find and retain work. This view was shared by people taking part in the National Survey of Adults with Learning Difficulties (Emerson et al 2005). They asked all the people who were currently unemployed why they did not have a job. 62% said this was because they could not get work, or nobody would give them a job. When asked if they would like a

INTELLECTUAL DISABILITY AND SOCIAL INCLUSION

job, 65% of this group said yes (Emerson et al 2005:51). Having now experienced a positive work environment, Mark's attitude towards employment has completely changed:

> 'I would be devastated unemployed, because I was unemployed for months, looking for work and dozens of interviews.'

Many people with intellectual disabilities fear that employers will not give them a job because of negative attitudes about the ability and capability of disabled people. Jeanette, who has worked at the café for two years, thinks that firms won't take on people with intellectual disabilities because they

> 'don't want us working here . . . They might have a nasty attitude and be frightened of them or something.'

Jeanette's fear may well be true. The Disability Rights Commission survey of 1000 small businesses (DRC 2004) looked at some of the potential barriers to employing people with disabilities. Although 53% of small businesses surveyed had a positive attitude to the principle of employing people with disabilities and 85% of this group had in place flexible work policies, only 1% felt a disabled person would fit into their team.

After 2 years at the café, Jeanette is clear about the qualities she brings to the team:

> 'I work hard and smile a lot! I am like a bit of the furniture.'

Her colleague Mark can sell his attributes as an employee:

> 'I am well mannered, punctual, I get on with people straight away and I am polite.'

Mark and Jeanette have all the requisite qualities for good employees.

Toucan's approach ties into one of the main messages from the Working Group on Learning Disabilities and Employment:

> 'People with learning disabilities are citizens first and foremost . . . the responsibility to ensure that all people can enter the workforce is a community based responsibility – not simply for health and social care.'
>
> Department for Work and Pensions 2006:1

Supported employment projects must understand the need to engage with employers as key leaders in local communities, to challenge their attitudes and perceptions and to offer them information and guidance. Often small employers feel in a similar position to that of people with intellectual disabilities themselves, in relation to additional support and advisory services that are available to support employment for disabled people (Disability Rights Commission 2004).

The Working Group on Learning Disabilities and Employment states that often employers are left feeling less than confident that people with learning disabilities will be able to carry out the job (Department for Work and Pensions 2006:12). Jeanette thinks that there should be a course for employers run by people with learning disabilities:

Getting into employment

'We could train them up. They need to know about how fast or slowly people can work. They need to know about disabilities, if people have mood swings – what people can and cannot do.'

Specialist employment agencies are no different from generic employment agencies – they have to sell the people on their books and sell their skill at being able to support their job seekers. Holding 'employers breakfasts' has proved to be an effective way to showcase the skills that employees like Mark and Jeanette can offer. It can also reassure employers, by showing them the infrastructure and support mechanisms available to them and their potential employees. It would appear that, although employment projects like Toucan engage with the local Learning Disability Partnership Board, the route to paid employment for people is through spending as much time in communities with local businesses, as strategic planning meetings with social care professionals.

Funding for supported employment projects makes up a tiny percentage of the estimated £4 billion that is spent on people with intellectual disabilities in England (Beyer et al 2004). Whereas so much is spent on health and social care services, there is very little spending by comparison on supporting people with intellectual disabilities to achieve employment. In my experience, employment projects often only receive a small amount of funding from the local authority for their work. Most of their money and much of their time is spent bidding for grants and awards.

In addition to forging alliances with local businesses, Toucan has come to appreciate the value of partnership working with families and carers. They feel that there is often a negative perception about families, and they can be viewed as reluctant to support their family member with an intellectual disability into employment. Toucan sees parents in the forefront of pushing for paid employment for people with intellectual disabilities. Toucan's Management Committee is led by a parent of a young adult with intellectual disabilities, and over the years they have supported an active parents group that is fully engaged in ensuring people with intellectual disabilities get local jobs. The parents see it as their role to represent Toucan at the intellectual disability Partnership Board and push for more effective local partnerships between key stakeholders, like Job Centre Plus and the Learning and Skills Council.

Ultimately, employees like Mark and Jeanette want exactly the same things from their jobs as the rest of the working population – money and the independence it brings. Jeanette wanted a job:

'because I wanted to have money on my own. I wanted my own money so I could save up for my holiday, get a new flat and things that I liked. I wanted to go out into the community.'

For Mark, he wanted to be more independent and be:

'like any other person coming and going to work.'

CONCLUSION

There are still many obstacles which continue to prevent people with intellectual disabilities from playing a full and active part in their communities and at work.

People have mostly been separated from their communities by long-stay hospitals, segregated schooling and continue to experience separate activities. This has led, and continues to engender, a lack of understanding about the contribution that people can make and about their capabilities and aspirations. Against this background, it is important that employment is not viewed as a means to an end in itself, but as a vital factor in building healthy, inclusive communities. If people with intellectual disabilities are excluded from opportunities to work they cannot fully participate in society. Supporting people into work can contribute significantly to fostering social inclusion and involvement of people in their communities.

It is important therefore that both the local and national agendas in relation to employment and social inclusion address the needs of people with intellectual disabilities. If working and employment are part of healthy communities, then resources must be allocated to ensuring that people with intellectual disabilities do not experience further social isolation, poverty and ill-health such as that associated with lack of employment in the general population.

There is a role for all of us working in this field to celebrate the success of stories like those told by Bev, Jeanette and Mark, not only within the circle of family and friends, but within the wider community as well.

REFERENCES

Beyer S, Grove B, Schneider J et al 2004 Working Lives: the role of day centres in supporting people with learning disabilities into employment (Department for Work and Pensions Research Report 2003). Corporate Document Services, Leeds.

Department for Work and Pensions 2002 Pathways to work: helping people into employment. HMSO, London.

Department for Work and Pensions 2003 Pathways to work: the government's response and action plan. HMSO, London.

Department for Work and Pensions 2006 Improving working opportunities for people with learning disabilities. A report to ministers and the learning disability task force. HMSO, London.

Department of Health 2001 Valuing People: A new strategy for learning disability of the 21st century. CM 5086.

Disability Rights Commission 2004 Getting into work – my rights. http://www. drc_gb.org/your_rights/employment/ getting_info_work_-_my_rights.aspx.

Disability Rights Commission 2005 Small employers attitudes to disability. http://www.drc-gb.org// library/research/empoyment/ small_employers_attitudes_to.aspx.

Disability Rights Commission 2006 Your rights at work: a guide for people with learning disabilities and their employers. http://www.drc_gb.org/your_rights/ employment/getting_info_work_-_my_ rights.aspx.

Emerson E, Malam S, Davies I, Spencer K 2005 Adults with learning difficulties in England. Government Statistical Service, Health and Social Care Information Centre.

Grove B, Mackintosh B 2005 Framework for developing employment strategy, valuing people support team. Institute for Applied Health and Social Policy, King's College London. http:// valuingpeople.gov.uk/dynamic/ valuing people.22.jsp.

Kennedy J, Poll C, Sanderson H 2004 Community connecting: discussion paper. http://www.in-control.org.uk/ pages-dev/in-search-upload.php.

King's Fund 1984 An ordinary working life: vocational services for people with mental handicap.

National Development Team 2007 Micro Enterprises. http://www.ndt.org.uk/ projectsN/ME.htm#wime.

Poll C 2005 Small Sparks how–to guide. http://www.in-control.org.uk/pages-dev/in-search-upload.php.

Prime Minister's Strategy Unit 2005 Prime Minister's Strategy Unit report to transform the life chances of disabled people. Cabinet Office, London.

Accessing further education

Jackie Martin

INTRODUCTION

This chapter considers issues in relation to inclusion in further education for adults with an intellectual disability. Adults with an intellectual disability were interviewed to ascertain their views on and experience of further education. Two organisations worked with me on this project. Positive Futures is an organisation which supports adults with an intellectual disability to access community facilities. Speaking Up is an Advocacy project for adults with an intellectual disability. Both organisations are based in Nottinghamshire. I gained access to both groups by approaching the organisation, explained that I wanted to interview adults with an intellectual disability for the purpose of writing this project. Staff within both organisations then asked people who they worked with if they would be interested in being interviewed by me about their experiences of going to college.

The result was that a group of people from Positive Futures were interested and willing to talk to me and a couple of individuals from Speaking Up were willing to do so. Consent was therefore gained by proxy with key staff members acting as gatekeepers for the project.

OBJECTIVES

The objectives of this chapter are:

- To report on a project that involved service users' perspectives of accessing further education
- To offer a theoretical framework upon which to understand the views expressed in this chapter
- To share some recommendations for professionals based on the views of service users involved in this project

The group I met at Positive Futures was a reference group who meet regularly to consider different types of information and feed back to the Positive Futures organisation upon whether the information they look at is accessible or not. I joined this group for a session as a guest and the group chose to speak to me as a group rather than be interviewed separately. The day I joined the group there were five people present, three men and two women. I did not meet with a group at Speaking Up, but met with two individuals who I interviewed separately. With all the interviews, I initially framed the questions in the same way for all interviewees, but if they weren't understood, I re-worded them. Not all the interviews kept strictly to the questions as some of the questions raised powerful experiences and it was appropriate when this happened to deviate from the schedule to acknowledge the importance of the experience for the person being interviewed.

The people interviewed attended different colleges and it has not been the purpose of this chapter to analyse the practice of any one college, but to find common themes in the experience of those interviewed, regardless of which college they attended.

THEORETICAL UNDERPINNING OF THE EXPERIENCE OF ADULTS WITH AN INTELLECTUAL DISABILITY

Thompson's (1998) PCS analysis describes three levels within which people are situated and experience oppression. In his analysis there are three levels:

- Personal
- Cultural
- Structural

Each of these levels operate separately but they are also interrelated. At the personal (P) level people have individual thoughts, feelings and prejudices which influence how they act towards others. In the PCS analysis, the personal level (P) is embedded in the cultural level (C). The cultural level refers to the way people live in a particular social group. The cultural level is in turn embedded in the structural level (S). Thompson states:

'The S level comprises the macro-level influences and constraints of the various social, political and economic aspects of the contemporary social order.'

Thompson 1998:16

Riddell (1996) has stated that for those who identify with the disability movement:

'the central justification of theory is its ability to promote social change.'

Riddell 1996:91

I am using Thompson's PCS analysis because it has the ability to promote social change, if it correctly understood. Change can be achieved in service provision when peoples' experiences of current services are understood and this understanding is used to develop them. I am not a disabled person and therefore do not pretend to have experienced the same things as disabled people. However, it has been my privilege to have been in employment which has brought me into contact with adults with an intellectual disability for a number of years and I have witnessed how they have been treated both by people and by systems. I have taken from this experience the conviction that social change is needed. I have come to understand the experience of individuals through the analysis of structural oppression. Structural oppression is the expression of the idea that individuals are oppressed through social processes and this is explored in Thompson's analysis.

As according to Riddell the disability movement claims that the central justification for theory is its ability to promote social change, this chapter will endeavour to apply the PCS analysis to understand the responses to the interviews and propose lessons to be learnt from them.

Paulo Friere stated:

'There is no such thing as a neutral education process. Education either functions as an instrument that is used to facilitate the integration of the young into the logic of the present system and bring about conformity to it or it becomes the practice of freedom. Education then becomes the means by which men and women deal critically and creatively with reality and discover how to participate in the transformation of the world.'

Friere 1972:56

If education is seen in this way, it provides a context in which to understand the experiences of adults with an intellectual disability. If education is a social process through which conformity to social order is reinforced or freedom is attained, then it has a role far beyond that of any curriculum and its stated intellectual outcomes. It also is identified as part of the societal processes which form part of the S level of Thompson's PCS analysis. The way colleges organise themselves and the wider policy and political frameworks which inform this provides us with an understanding of the S level, whereas the way people behave within them provides us with an understanding of the C and P levels.

RESEARCH AND INTELLECTUALLY DISABLED PEOPLE

The interviewees were asked about their experience of further education. This is of course only one aspect of peoples' lives and can only be seen as providing a very partial picture of the experience of adults with an intellectual disability, but there are lessons to be learnt which will provide valuable learning for all who support adults with an intellectual disability in all aspects of their lives.

INVOLVING PEOPLE WITH AN INTELLECTUAL DISABILITY IN RESEARCH

Porter & Lacey (2005:91) provide a useful summary of challenges for the researcher to overcome when working with adults with an intellectual disability:

- The agenda is meaningful for the person, or indeed set by them
- A relationship is established by which people feel empowered to have a view and time and opportunity are given
- The context in which the research takes place reduces the cognitive and linguistic demands of participation
- A systematic approach is taken to verifying the views

These points are important as to address them is to attempt to work in a way which is not in itself oppressive, but rather gives people the opportunity to voice their opinions and tell their stories. The agenda and interview schedule were shared with both projects prior to the interviews and the workers then approached people they worked with to take part based on this knowledge. I did not have access to the interviewees prior to the interviews, but in all cases, except for Amanda (who chose to be on her own), the worker from the project was present during the interviews and they were well known to the interviewees. All interviews took place at the premises used by the projects and so were familiar to the interviewees and the questions were rephrased or repeated if this was needed. The interviews were written up and the contents verified by the project workers with the interviewees and the results then fed back to me. There were some matters of fact which I had misunderstood in one of the interviews which I amended when informed of this.

Porter & Lacey (2005:86) state '...a fundamental role for research is to bring about changes in policy and practices through revealing how lives are constrained by the acts of oppressors'. The project outlined in this chapter was participatory in the way interviewees were consulted about how they wanted to be referred to, the use that was to be made of their interviews, the verification of what they wanted to say after it was written up. The interviewees were not consulted about the formation of the interview questions. The workers who supported them from both agencies were consulted about the interview questions as they rightly wanted to be sure of the intention of the project. This fact does not negate the relevance or legitimacy of the project as its aim and the motivation of the agencies and the interviewees does comply fully with Porter & Lacey's 'fundamental role' as detailed above. People took part with the project because they wanted people who work with people with an intellectual disability to read about their experiences and for practice and systems to change as a result.

The members of the group from Positive Futures all said that they would like their names to be recorded in this chapter, so they were: Helen Goddard, Roger Grange, Nicki Clarke, Leigh Mekin and Richard Turner.

The two individuals from Speaking Up were Louise and Amanda Platts. Louise has Down's syndrome and asked that she be referred to as 'Louise'. She also asked that the readers of this chapter be told that she has been married for 3 years at the time of being interviewed (2006). Amanda was the only person of the seven people that I interviewed who has a mild intellectual disability. The results of the interviews are indicated below quantitatively with the numbers referring to the number of interviewees who responded in the way indicated. As the interviews were semi-structured and the interviewees were able to share their experiences as well as provide an answer to the questions these experiences are also recorded. This has resulted in some qualitative results being detailed as Louise and Amanda in particular had stories to tell which they thought important to be included in this chapter. This approach of recording quantitative and qualitative findings may not be very neat, but it is consistent with the stated aim of the project to share experience and for this to change practice. An aim which would be very difficult to achieve with quantitative data alone.

FINDINGS

The interview questions are indicated together with the responses which were given to them in Table 11.1.

Table 11.1 **Interview questions and responses**

Do you enjoy going to college?

Yes	6
No	1

What do you enjoy about it?

Meeting people	1
Learning new skills	3
Eating the meals in the canteen	1
A computer course	1
I didn't like anything at all	1

What would you change about college if you could?

I would have smaller groups	3
I would like to have somewhere to smoke	1
I would like to be listened to more by the tutor	1
I would like the bullying to stop	
I would like more space in facilities, in the accessible toilets for example	1

What do you want to learn at college? Is college helping you with this?

Each interviewee had a different response to this question:	
Geography	No, not helping
Working with computers	No, not helping
First Aid	No, not helping
Drama	No longer attending college, so not applicable
How to get a job	No, not helping
How to deal with bullying	No, not helping
Makaton (simplified signed English)	No, not helping
About car engines	Yes, I am learning this at college

Is your course only for people with a learning disability?

Just for people with a learning disability	5
For disabled and non-disabled people	1 (car mechanics)
I have attended courses just for people with a learning disability and courses which are for disabled and non-disabled people	1 (photography was the inclusive course)

Continued

Table 11.1 Interview questions and responses (*Continued*)	
Would you like to do a course at college which is for anyone, not just people with a learning disability? Why?	
I would prefer to be in a course which isn't just for people with a learning disability	2
I would like to attend a mixture of some courses just for people with a learning disability and some for other people as well as people with a learning disability	3
I would prefer courses just for people with a learning disability	2

The two people who said they would prefer inclusive classes added that they might need support to access these. One of the people who said he likes to have a mixture of both said that one thing he did like about the inclusive class is that he mixed with people his own age rather than be put in a group which covered school leavers up to older people. The two people who said they preferred groups just for people with an intellectual disability cited the fact that they can talk more openly about issues such as bullying and that people might be more inclined to help each other in a segregated group. The two people who said they preferred groups just for people with an intellectual disability had not attended college courses which were inclusive. The person who had attended inclusive classes said that he preferred a mixture of the two. Louise thought that classes should be mixed although her experience had only been of segregated courses. She wouldn't attend college again as she didn't enjoy her time there, but if she did it would be to learn more about being independent and going into the community. Amanda attended courses which were just for adults with an intellectual disability as well as those that which were for non-adults with an intellectual disability. Amanda said she likes attending both types of courses; she enjoys the content more of the non-intellectually disabled groups but enjoys supporting adults with greater needs than her in the specialist provision (just for adults with an intellectual disability). Although she enjoys attending both types of group, Amanda believes that groups should be mixed as this 'educates' people without an intellectual disability if they attend inclusive groups. Amanda did not have support at college and found it difficult at first without support in the non-specialist courses as she was unclear what was expected of her. Amanda reflected that she was bullied while she was at school, and while she hadn't experienced bullying for at least 11 years, this experience made her uncertain about mixing and this has impacted on how she felt about attending non-specialist courses.

DISCUSSION OF VIEWS EXPRESSED

Although a variety of views were expressed by the interviewees, common themes are elicited. Most people stated that they enjoyed college. There was not a consensus about whether inclusion is desirable on college courses. However, although the principle of inclusion was discussed, only two of the people interviewed had been given the opportunity to attend courses which were open to non-adults with an intellectual disability, so five people's opinions were not based on experience of inclusive courses. From the group interview, it is interesting to note that the only person who thought the college was helping him with what he really wanted to learn is the person who attended an inclusive course. The reasons given for enjoying college were social, or having the opportunity to undertake craft activities. Both of the people who had attended inclusive as well as segregated courses said they enjoyed attending both types of courses and felt they had benefited from attending the mainstream courses. The main reasons that were expressed for preferring segregated courses were in terms of fear of not having enough support and not being able to talk openly about issues such as bullying.

The experience of bullying was a common theme both at college and before college. With the people interviewed, this was bullying by non-disabled adults or children. The two people who had attended inclusive courses did not report this as part of their experience on these courses, although one of them had feared that this might happen.

The dissatisfaction expressed in relation to segregated courses was the size of the groups in terms of there being too many people for the tutor to support, the groups being too noisy to concentrate in and the classes being for all ages. For the youngest person interviewed, who had only left school a few years previously, the fact that no-one his own age was in the segregated groups was a real issue for him.

BARRIERS TO ACCESSING FURTHER EDUCATION

Two-tier system

One of the most striking aspects of the interviews was the sense that although all of the people interviewed had attended further education colleges which are accessible to everyone, the courses that most of them attended were not inclusive and they had not all been given the opportunity to access truly inclusive courses. Although they had attended courses in a building where other people attended courses which were not segregated, they were not given the opportunity to access these. In fact, in one case, it was the attitude of some of these non-disabled people who prevented further attendance at college. There seems to be a two-tier further education system taking place with some adults with an intellectual disability and this is an example of structural oppression at the S level in Thompson's analysis. One tier is for adults with an intellectual disability and the other is for non-adults with an intellectual disability. Sometimes, as shown in the interviews, adults with an intellectual disability do access the other tier. This was in fact the experience of Amanda, who has a mild intellectual disability, but only of one other person who accessed the car mechanics course. There often does not seem to be any way for adults with a moderate or a severe intellectual disability to progress from one tier to the next. There seems to be a structural barrier between the two and it is very difficult to navigate across it. This barrier seems to be the result of how some further education colleges are currently structured. There may be colleges where this is not the case and where adults can progress from one level to another, but this does not seem to be the case for those interviewed. The responses to the question asking what courses people would like to do that they do not do currently indicated a number of courses which would almost certainly be offered to non-disabled students but the interviewees did not feel that the colleges were helping them to access these.

Bullying

The second most striking factor which creates a very real barrier to people is the experience of bullying. The discrimination experienced by adults with an intellectual disability is widely acknowledged, but the power of the interviewees telling their own stories really emphasised what a huge barrier this is to them. This is structural oppression as experienced at the P level in Thompson's analysis. The intellectual disability of the interviewees will not be cited as a barrier to inclusion in further education. It is not their ignorance, but the ignorance and prejudice of others expressed through bullying that has created this barrier. A barrier of fear seems a huge barrier to tackle as even if bullying is appropriately challenged (when it is known about), the fear left by previous bullying can have a really disabling effect on a person.

POLICY DIRECTIVES

Further education

The Further Education and Higher Education Act 1992 created the Further Education Funding Council (FEFC) and colleges were directed to have regard to services to people with intellectual difficulties. Progress in relation to this was reviewed in the report *Inclusive Learning* (FEFC 1996). The report discusses an inclusive learning philosophy. It states:

'There is a world of difference between, on the one hand, offering
courses of education and training and then giving some students who
have intellectual difficulties some additional human or physical aids
to gain access to these courses and, on the other hand, redesigning
the very processes of learning, assessment and organisation so as to
fit the objectives and learning styles of students. But only the second
philosophy can claim to be inclusive, to have as its central purpose
the opening of opportunity to those whose disability means that they
learn differently from others. It may mean introducing new content into
courses or it may mean differentiated access to the same content or both.'
Further Education Funding Council 1996:4

The experience of the adults interviewed seems to suggest that the first approach is sometimes adopted, but there is no evidence of the second approach being adopted. As we have already intimated, this is an expression of oppression at the S level in Thompson's analysis as this is about how organisations are run and how that excludes people. It may be the case that there are truly inclusive courses, as defined above, but the interviews suggest that, if there are, they are not the experience of all. It was not the remit of this chapter to look at the practice of individual further education colleges, but there are some questions which each college could ask itself when reviewing their inclusion of people with an intellectual disability. Firstly, is it possible to progress from specialist provision to inclusive courses? If not, why not? Is it the assessment practices that prevent inclusion; for example, are all assessments written assessments? If this is the case, is there another way of assessing people, maybe through practical demonstration or verbally? There will be courses where written assessment may be essential, but there are also many where this is how people are assessed, but this could be done in a different way. If adults with an intellectual disability were able to access courses where they could obtain a qualification, this may have a positive impact on their desire for employment.

A SUGGESTED MODEL OF INCLUSIVE FURTHER EDUCATION

It is not the intention of this chapter to criticise further education colleges as there may well be colleges which are offering excellent courses which are fully inclusive. It is the purpose to ascertain how such courses may be recognised though and also how those that are not truly inclusive may also be recognised. An inclusive course would have systems in place whereby applications are accepted from disabled as well as non-disabled applicants. It would have teaching which was intelligible to all the students, expressed in language which is understood by all students. It would have means of assessing students in ways which do not rely on written skills and would test understanding or skill acquisition as appropriate by verbal feedback or demonstration of skills, whichever is appropriate. A fully inclusive course would not use the acquisition of written skills as a barrier to accessing it when writing is just a means to an end and assessment can be made in other ways. A fully inclusive course would not just mix intellectually disabled and non-disabled people in the same building, but in the same classroom. It would also offer support if this was needed individually. If all of the adults interviewed had a positive experience of accessing community resources if they were appropriately supported, then this could be replicated in further education.

The Valuing People White Paper (Department of Health 2001) has 'rights, independence, choice and inclusion' as its four key principles. In light of the experiences shared in the interviews, it is not hard to see that it is difficult for adults with an intellectual disability to realise these principles in their experience.

LEARNING POINTS FOR PROFESSIONALS WISHING TO SUPPORT ADULTS WITH AN INTELLECTUAL DISABILITY TO ACCESS FURTHER EDUCATION

Education is a valuable part of everyone's life and it is vital that adults with an intellectual disability are given the same opportunities to access education as every other citizen. However, there are key question to be asked about the value of some courses for people. The principles of care planning should be fully adhered to in that care planning should follow and be based on an assessment of needs (Department of Health 1990, para 3.24). The actual needs which the college course is to meet should be considered carefully and the question should be posed as to whether the course does in fact meet these needs rather than being a way to occupy someone during the day.

It often seems impossible for professionals to change structural barriers, but unless people challenge structures by asking questions of those who uphold them, then nothing will ever change. If you as a professional think that the college is not including adults with an intellectual disability in the way defined above by the FEFC, then it is part of your responsibility to challenge this. Also, it is important that where you see that colleges are including people fully, you pass on your comments regarding this as too many people only comment where there is a difficulty. According to Thompson, social workers have a duty to challenge oppression (1992, cited in Thompson 1997:11). He writes:

'There is no middle ground; intervention either adds to oppression (or at least condones it) or goes some small way towards easing or breaking such oppression. In this respect, the political slogan 'If you are not part of the solution, you must be part of the problem' is particularly accurate. An awareness of the socio-political context is necessary in order to prevent becoming (or remaining) part of the problem.'

If an adult with an intellectual disability is unable to access courses which s/he would benefit from because the college structures prevent it, workers supporting them have a duty to challenge this. They may or may not be able to change anything for the person they are working with, but if systems are constantly being challenged, then there is more likelihood that they will be reviewed.

In relation to bullying, professionals need to understand the impact that this has on the lives of intellectually disabled adults as is more than adequately evidenced by Louise's interview. Bullying is not a trivial manner and instances need to be taken seriously and addressed through the appropriate channels. This might mean working with the college in relation to educating individuals or it might even mean a Safeguarding Adults (adult protection) investigation.

SUMMARY

While the interviews revealed different experiences and different views about the desirability of inclusion in relation to further education, some themes were constant. All interviewees valued either studying or learning skills alongside non-adults with an intellectual disability if the experience was a positive one for them in terms of not being bullied and receiving adequate support.

It is not enough for professionals to be committed to the idea of inclusion; they must understand the barriers to it and how to begin to tackle them. In order to do this, an understanding has to be gained of the personal and structural discrimination that people will face. Just as importantly, professionals must know the adults they are supporting or assessing well enough to work with them on providing the right type of support they need. It is not acceptable to set someone up to fail, by presenting them with situations for which they are unprepared.

Louise saw a role for colleges in helping her to be more independent and learn about going into the community. Perhaps her vision is of services which work together to enable people to realise their citizen rights. Perhaps if colleges could work with families, housing providers or tenancy support services and with the adults with an intellectual disability themselves to help them learn the skills they want for accessing leisure and employment then inclusion would be one step nearer. This may well already be happening in some colleges, which would be excellent, but it does not appear to be the experience of the adults interviewed for this chapter.

Thompson's PCS analysis which we looked at earlier provides us with a way of understanding that people are oppressed in different ways through their direct contact with people (as in bullying), through cultural, or through structural forces such as the way education is organised. To remind ourselves of Riddell's claim that those who align themselves with the disability movement see the central justification for theory to be to effect social change is to remind ourselves of our responsibility if we work with and support adults with an intellectual disability.

It is a real privilege to play some part in the inclusion of an intellectually disabled adult in society. To see them learning new skills, forming new relationships or just having a good time is seeing things as they should be, but at the moment it is not everyone's experience. It is to this end that we should all strive.

ACKNOWLEDGEMENTS

My thanks to Marie O'Sullivan from Speaking Up and Jim Broughton from Positive Futures for their support as well as to the interviewees who are named in the way they chose to be in this chapter.

REFERENCES

Department of Health 1990 Community Care in the next decade and beyond: policy guidance. Department of Health, London.

Department of Health 2001 Valuing People: a new strategy for learning disability for the 21st century. Department of Health, London.

Further Education Funding Council 1996 Inclusive learning: principles and recommendations – a summary of the findings of the learning difficulties committee. FEFC, Coventry.

Friere P 1972 Pedagogy of the oppressed. Penguin, Harmondsworth.

Porter J, Lacey P 2005 Researching learning difficulties, a guide for practitioners. Sage.

Riddell S 1996 Theorising special educational needs in a changing political climate. In: Barton L (ed) Disability and society, emerging issues and insights. Longman, London and New York.

Thompson N 1997 Anti-discriminatory practice. Macmillan, Basingstoke.

Thompson N 1998 Promoting equality, challenging discrimination and oppression in the human services. Palgrave.

Accessing further education

Getting equal housing

Steven Rose

INTRODUCTION

'An Englishman's home is his castle' is an old adage that sums up the importance that our society places on the individual's home. Having one's own home, for most of us, ranks alongside our partners, children, job, good health and social life as one of the fundamentally most important things in our lives.

Most adult members of the general population either own their own home (a small proportion owning two or more), or rent their home from their local council, a housing association or private landlord. There are of course a significant minority of people who do not fit into these categories, including a very small number of adults who continue to live with their parents for many years after attaining adulthood, members of the armed forces, members of religious orders, students and some older people in sheltered accommodation or residential or nursing care. However, these individuals have usually either chosen a life pursuit that dictates the type of accommodation that they occupy or they are at a particular stage in their life, e.g. students or elderly people. Of course most students will go on to have their own home and most elderly people in care have previously owned a home or been a tenant.

Contrast the model of housing enjoyed by most members of the general population with the experience of people with intellectual disabilities and a very different picture begins to emerge. There is no overall statistic that identifies exactly where each adult with an intellectual disability lives. However, there have been a number of recent studies that are relevant and a summary of these is set out below.

Between July 2003 and October 2004 the first ever national survey of adults with intellectual disabilities was completed by a research team made up of BMRB Social Research, Professor Eric Emerson, from the Institute for Health Research at Lancaster University, and Central England People First (Emerson et al 2005). The team interviewed 2898 people with intellectual disabilities who were at least 16 years old. This work produced data on where people surveyed with intellectual disabilities were actually living (Fig. 12.1).

An examination of the technical appendices to the National Survey reveals the distribution of those people with intellectual disabilities who were in some sort of care (Table 12.1).

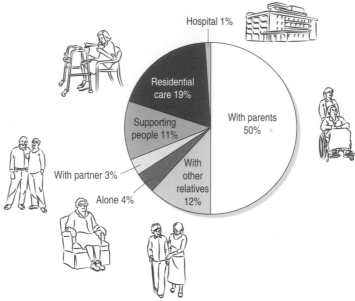

Where people were living

Hospital 1%

Residential care 19%

Supporting people 11%

With partner 3%

Alone 4%

With other relatives 12%

With parents 50%

Fig. 12.1 Where people were living (Emerson et al 2005). Copyright © 2008. Re-used with the permission of The Information Centre. All rights reserved.

Table 12.1 Distribution of people with intellectual disability who are in some sort of care. Copyright © 2008. Re-used with the permission of The Information Centre. All rights reserved

Sector	Source	Year	Estimated number
NHS hospital beds	NHS Hospital Activity Statistics	2002/3	3003
NHS residential care beds	NHS Hospital Activity Statistics	2002/3	2777
Registered residential care homes	NCSC and LA Residential Care Statistical Returns	2002/3	46356
Supporting People programmes	ODPM		27452
Total			79588

Source: technical appendix to National Survey, Emerson et al (2005), available via http://www.ic.nhs.uk/pubs/learndiff2004

A collective review of the recent information for England is shown in Table 12.2.

As stated above there is a significant difference between accommodation options for people with intellectual disabilities and most of the rest of the population. This difference goes way beyond the type of accommodation occupied and includes the facts that most people in residential care and supported living live in groups and very few live with a partner.

Table 12.2 Collective review of the recent information for England		
	Approx. %	*Numbers*
Adults living in the parental home	49	90000
In residential care homes	32	60000
In supported housing shared and s/c*	12	22000
In adult placement	3	5000
In NHS care	4	7000
Long-stay hospital		1000
Total	100%	185000

*More recent Supporting People (SP) figures now suggest higher numbers – nearer 30000, but this may reflect some double counting of registered care homes, additional SP services and more comprehensive recording (Harker 2003).

WHAT IS THE WAY FORWARD?

It is usually relatively easy, as I have done above, to identify a problem. It is often much more difficult to accurately pinpoint the precise cause of the problem and even more difficult to find a solution to the problem. A number of innovative individuals and organisations have begun to address inequality in housing options for people with intellectual disabilities. The remainder of this chapter is devoted to case studies from five sources:

- Housing Options
- The 'in Control' project
- Progress Care Housing Association
- Advance Housing and Care
- The Association for Supported Living

Each of the case studies illustrates how an individual(s) with intellectual disabilities has been supported to 'Get Equal Housing'. Some of them are examples of what was achieved more than a decade ago. These case studies can be replicated elsewhere and each of the organisations cited are available to help more and more people with intellectual disabilities to 'Get Equal Housing'. This chapter does not attempt to offer detailed advice on how to set up the schemes illustrated in the case studies.

HOUSING OPTIONS

In 1996 a report *Ownership Options* was commissioned by two housing associations and published by the National Housing Federation. It provided six detailed case studies on examples of home ownership for someone with an intellectual disability. The report raised much interest. It soon became clear that there was a considerable demand for information and advice and the Housing Options service was established.

It created not only interest but contributed toward a revolution in the way of thinking about services for people with intellectual disabilities. There has been a culture of professionals deciding what is best for you. Housing Options listened to what people said they wanted. The most influential statement of this was in 'Valuing People' (Department of Health 2001):

> 'People with learning disabilities can live successfully in different types of housing...the full range of tenures, including home ownership.'

The other theme was the importance of helping people to plan ahead. The response from Housing Options was to try to:

- Think seriously about a wider range of options
- Help people to plan ahead
- Develop practicable solutions

The job now is to make it all happen and there is a big gap between policy hopes and the real experience of most people with intellectual disabilities.

Case study 12.1   Rebecca's story

Rebecca lived in some form of residential care since she was 8. At 26 she became the part owner of a bungalow in a village in Lincolnshire. She has very little language although she finds other ways to communicate. Brain damaged at birth, she suffers severe epilepsy and is unable to walk.

Rebecca's residential care home, run by Barnardos, was closing. This prompted a review of the next steps for Rebecca. Rebecca, her parents and the residential care project all agreed that a large scale residential care setting was no longer a good or suitable place for Rebecca. She was not participating in the social activities that can be one of the benefits of being part of a large community. She had become somewhat withdrawn. Whenever she came home to stay with her parents she became very distressed on being taken back to the residential care project where she was clearly no longer happy. It was agreed that the best thing would be to try and combine a personal care package for Rebecca with a degree of independence somewhere much closer to her parents. Rebecca's parents knew that they themselves could not provide the kind of constant and intensive support that Rebecca needed, nor was their own home very suitable. The problem of finding somewhere sufficiently close to the parents so that they could again play a bigger part in supporting their daughter was solved by them acquiring a plot of land adjacent to their existing home and having a property built.

Rebecca's parents could afford to contribute to the plot of land but could not afford to construct a new house suitable for Rebecca and the support staff that she would always need. They obtained a list of local housing associations from the National Housing Federation. They wrote to a number explaining they were seeking a means of providing a specially adapted bungalow for their disabled daughter. The Chief Executive of Longhurst Housing Association eventually replied in a very positive and encouraging way pledging his association's support to 'find a way'. The constant support of staff at Longhurst has been central to providing the housing and Rebecca's parents speak very highly of the help they have received.

The initial proposal was that Rebecca's parents would sell their plot of land to the association which would construct a bungalow to rent designed around Rebecca's needs. Although Rebecca's parents were prepared to sell the plot at less than cost in order to make the project possible, the Housing Corporation, who provide housing associations with the necessary grant, rejected a rented scheme as poor value for money.

The Housing Association then came up with the idea of using the low cost home ownership programme instead and a local builder completed the construction of a purpose-designed, three-bedroom bungalow for Rebecca. Rebecca's parents took out the mortgage for the purchased share of the property which is repaid from Income Support for Mortgage Interest and rent is covered by Housing Benefit. (The financial arrangements can be complex and information is available about this on the Housing Options website.) Rebecca's sister sums up the change like this: 'Every time I think about her being in the bungalow the word 'momentous' always springs to mind. I cannot believe that it is now reality.' Most people would not appreciate the sheer significance of such an event. This case study first appeared in *Ownership Options* (1996) – author Nigel King.

'IN CONTROL'

In June 2003 the Valuing People Support Team, Mencap, Paradigm, Helen Sanderson Associates and the North West Training & Development Team came together to launch 'in Control'. The objective of 'in Control' is the complete transformation of social care into a system of self-directed support. Since then 'in Control' has worked to pilot some of the key elements of self-directed support, to build a wider alliance to support self-directed support and to recommend changes in local and national policy and practice. By 2006 when the first 18 months of 'in Control' was evaluated (Poll et al 2006) it was already clear that self-directed support was one effective way for people to get equal housing. Clive's story is just one example.

Case study 12.2   Clive's story: Clive's main objective in directing his support was to move from the group home to his own place

Clive lives in his own home in Bristol. He first heard about 'in Control' at a *People First* meeting. He thought it sounded 'all right'.

At that time, about 2 years ago, Clive was living in a group home with six other people. He didn't like living there. The people he shared the home with often argued. This made the house quite noisy. Once, he was hit with a snooker cue by another resident. Other residents often used to 'tell him off'. These were just some of the problems that Clive faced in the group home. He had to go into the office to talk to staff about these problems. It used to make him very nervous and the problems never seemed to be sorted out.

Continued

Case study 12.2   Clive's story: Clive's main objective in directing his support was to move from the group home to his own place—cont'd

Clive needed to take quite a few tablets for health reasons. In the home, he always had someone watching him take his tablets. Clive would say 'I'm not a baby, I'm an adult' and the staff would reply that they had to watch him to make sure he took his tablets. This made him feel angry.

He had to go to bed at 10 p.m. during the week and at 11 p.m. at weekends. He wasn't happy about being told when to go to bed. In fact, all in all, Clive was 'fed up' with where he was living, who he had to live with and the support he received from staff. He was sharing a home with people who needed 24-hour support, 7 days a week, and he didn't need this. So, when he heard about 'in Control', he thought that this was his chance to be more in control of his life and to make some changes.

Clive found the first 'in Control' meeting he went to 'nerve wracking'. He was more confident at the second meeting and his confidence steadily grew. Clive's family is important to him, so when he started planning for his future, he really wanted them to be involved. His Mum and his two brothers, Paul and Mark, supported him to put his plan together. Even though Mark lives in Bradford and Paul lives in Canada, they attended meetings, telephoned and sent emails to support Clive.

Clive also did some training to become a trainer of person-centred planning. He also had support from Alison, a support broker, and his social worker. With everyone's support and his training, Clive found that he was now making decisions about what he wanted to see changed in his life.

Plans were agreed, money was allocated and Clive set about looking for a new home. His brother, Paul, came over from Canada and together they looked at quite a few houses.

Eventually, they found the right house in a quiet residential area of Bristol. Paul decided he would like to buy the house and Clive was happy for Paul to become his landlord. Clive moved into his new home in June 2005. Clive says 'moving out is pretty good'. He says he is happier than before. No-one watches him take his tablets. His support staff still asks him if he has remembered to take them but the support is on his terms. He chooses when he goes to bed.

When his brothers phone him, he answers the phone himself now instead of the staff. Clive has learnt how to use his own washing machine and is proud of the plants he has planted in his own garden. If he has problems now, the staff sort them out. If he has any problems with the staff, he can, as he says, 'sack them'! It took Clive a while to get used to being in control in this way, but now he is more confident and knows that things will change if he is not happy about anything.

However, as you would expect, not everything went smoothly. For example, there were problems sorting out benefit payments. In spite of support from relatives, support workers, the support broker and the

Citizens Advice Bureau, 3 months after moving into his new home, things still hadn't been sorted out. The benefits staff in the various departments and offices seemed unable or unwilling to deal with Clive's support staff when phoning on his behalf. Issues were often passed from one member of the benefits staff team to another each time they phoned.

But Clive is looking forward now. He would like to get a job (as long as he will be better off financially!). He would like to tell others about 'in Control'. He would like to do this so that more people can do what he has done.

PROGRESS CARE HOUSING ASSOCIATION

Formed in 1998 under the umbrella of Progress Housing Group, Progress Care Housing Association (PCHA) provides a specialist, supported housing management service. Currently managing 1700 units of accommodation in England and Scotland, the majority of the Association's housing stock is based on a shared, supported living model.

The Association's successful earlier work, in providing housing for people moving from long-stay institutional care, established it a reputation for the quick delivery of quality schemes. From the beginning PCHA has regarded partnership working as essential to providing independent living accommodation and it works with a large number of different purchasing and support-providing organisations.

PCHA's ethos is one of flexibility. It prides itself on providing housing solutions to meet the specific needs and requirements of people with mental health problems, intellectual difficulties and physical disabilities. In addition PCHA offers shared ownership as an alternative to renting accommodation. These schemes offer people with intellectual difficulties the opportunity to enjoy the benefits of home ownership.

PCHA is able to deliver a high quality service both because of its access to funding opportunities and its dedicated team of housing management officers, who work alongside a development team working solely on supported housing schemes. As a result the organisation has built up a wealth of knowledge and understanding of the needs of people with requiring support and is well placed to enable them to lead dignified and fulfilling lives.

Here are some examples of the ways that PCHA delivers results that make a real difference to lives:

- *In the beginning*. At the development stage PCHA explores with service commissioners, prospective tenants and their advisors exactly what they want and need. Behavioural problems can bring their own particular challenges, with solutions ranging from strengthened doors or walls and magnetic curtain tracking to sound-proofed walls and window safety filming.
- *Physical adaptations*. Ensuring that tenants' homes are fully accessible enhances independent living. New schemes will include appropriate adaptations, such as ramps, ceiling hoists, grab rails, internal wheelchair

access and specialist bathing equipment. However, just as importantly is helping tenants to live in their homes for as long as possible. To ensure this, a charge is included in the rent to carry out subsequent small-scale improvements and adaptations.

- *Secure tenancies.* Many of the people living in PCHA properties have, for the first time, security of tenure. This gives them homes of their own in which to develop living skills and to decorate as they wish. It is also an opportunity to become integrated into, and to contribute positively to, the local community, while forming new friendships and interests.

- *Empowering tenants.* Having a tenancy brings both rights and responsibilities. PCHA places great emphasis on making sure this message is understood, by producing information in varied, attractive formats, such as a video/DVD, pictorial tenancy agreement, tenant's handbook and information leaflets.

- *Involving tenants.* PCHA have an active tenant participation programme and have a dedicated tenant involvement officer to encourage this participation. PCHA aims to involve tenants in ways that best suits them. At one level this may be designing a front cover for a booklet, filling in a satisfaction survey or sending in a story for the tenant's newsletter. At another level it may be attending a tenant's meeting and commenting on the service PCHA provide or the contents of the next newsletter.

- *Specialist housing management service.* Flexibility remains the key word in PCHA's approach to housing management, although clear roles are established from the beginning between PCHA the service commissioners and support agencies through management and lease agreements. PCHA's expertise ensures that independent living is supported by the maximisation of eligible Housing Benefit income. While those tenant households that able to, are encouraged in their independence to manage their own home accounts for items like gardening services, utilities and window cleaning.

Case study 12.3 Jane's story

Jane moved from residential care to a Progress Care Housing bungalow two and half years ago. She lives there with two fellow tenants and has a team of three support workers who support her in developing her daily living skills.

Jane says that since she has lived in her new home she has learnt to cope with many different aspects of daily living, such as using the washing machine, hoovering, cleaning, accessing the community, and how to get along with people. She has found that communicating with people is the key to a happy house and ability to live together with others.

Jane told us that her support team had helped her to take holidays. Her first holiday was to a holiday camp not too far away because she hadn't taken a holiday for a long time and felt quite nervous about going away. All went well though and everyone had a great time. Since then Jane has been to London with a fellow tenant where she said they had a fantastic time but she has also built up the confidence to take other breaks independently.

Jane lives life to the full in other ways too. She attends a day service during the week where she undertakes lots of different activities, she is part of a catering group for which she gets paid and she also attends college to learn maths skills so that she can budget her finances. Jane also attends church and a bible class and is delighted to be able to go swimming again, an activity she hasn't been able to do for 15 years.

Jane said 'I think I'm enjoying my life to the full, however I'm always willing to try new activities put to me and I feel a lot more confident in myself and I love the town I now live in.'

ADVANCE HOUSING AND SUPPORT

Over the past nine years Oxford-based housing association Advance Housing and Support has helped over 274 people with intellectual difficulties or mental health problems move into their own properties on a shared ownership basis. In 2007 they plan to work with a further 85 people through the government HomeBuy scheme and a further 30 people through the family funded route.

Advance, set up 30 years ago to help sidelined disadvantaged people realise their potential as valued citizens, lobbied government to recognise the needs of disabled people, who weren't included in the original HomeBuy consultation document. The government's scheme was primarily targeted at streamlining the multi-faceted home ownership regime and providing a large amount of affordable housing for tenants and key workers.

The government aims to have helped some 100 000 households to own their own home by 2010, with HomeBuy, which will be used as a guide by the Housing Corporation as it consider bids for grants in the 2006–2008 Affordable Housing Programme. It streamlines the old system into three new projects: Social HomeBuy, aimed at social tenants; New Build HomeBuy, enabling people to buy a share in a newly built property; and Open Market HomeBuy, under which Advance will operate. Advance was the first provider to take advantage of HomeBuy and is now the acknowledged expert in the Shared Ownership sector. The Advance team support clients every step of the way, from getting grant aid to surveying and buying the house the clients choose. The help continues after the new owners move in, with Advance providing a support network and carrying out minor repairs and improvements.

Case study 12.4 Jeremy Court's story

Thousands of parents are facing the kind of dilemma which confronted Wiltshire couple Shirley and Nelson Court. Worried about providing a secure and stable future for their Down's Syndrome son Jeremy they had no idea where to turn, until they heard a chance remark about a charitable organisation which seemed to provide the answer they were searching for.

Continued

Getting equal housing

Case study 12.4 Jeremy Court's story—cont'd

When Nelson Court heard the name Advance mentioned during a meeting to discuss Jeremy's future plans, he went home and set to work.

He made a call to Advance's Head of Home Ownership Graeme Jackson and set in motion events which have changed their lives and that of their son Jeremy.

'Advance has taken a huge weight off our shoulders. That's the only way to describe what they have done for us' said Nelson, dad to 39-year-old Jeremy.

'Jeremy had been sharing a rented charity-run flat about 2 miles from our village of Purton. He had been reasonably settled there for the past 5 years then the place closed down and he had to come home' he explained.

Having Jeremy back at home where he had always lived before wasn't a disaster. A sociable and loving son he had his own room and enjoyed a loving relationship with his parents, but the future was what worried Nelson and Shirley.

'I'm almost 75, my wife almost 70 and there will come a time when we won't be able to care for Jeremy anymore. We needed to plan for that day and Advance has provided some of the answers we were looking for' said Nelson.

Through their innovative nationwide Shared Ownership housing scheme Advance offers people with intellectual disabilities or mental health problems the chance to choose their own home and own a large share of it, with Advance owning the remainder.

The Courts found Jeremy a small house nearby, Advance sent a surveyor to help assess it and any work needed. The Courts were only required to pay Stamp Duty and solicitors' fees.

'Everything went very smoothly, Advance were extremely good and helped us every step of the way. I didn't know that such a scheme as this existed but it is a very simple and effective idea.

'Jeremy's Income Support goes to pay the interest only mortgage which he has taken out and his Housing Benefit goes to pay the rental element which also covers maintenance. So Jeremy owns 65% of the house and Advance 35%' he explained.

In the 2 years since he moved into his house the Courts have watched their son blossom.

Jeremy will always need to be supported to live alone and has a team of three carers round the clock, paid for through the council funded system of Direct Payments, but for the first time he could relish the independence having his own home brought him.

'He is really still over the moon about it. Having his own space and some independence for the first time is very important to him. He can be by himself to listen to his music and watch his television, but we know he is safe and secure' said Nelson, who is very happy to have Jeremy home at weekends when they can enjoy outings to watch their local soccer team together.

THE ASSOCIATION FOR SUPPORTED LIVING

The Association for Supported Living is a not-for-profit association comprising support and housing providers, in England, providing supported living for people with intellectual disabilities. The purpose of the ASL is to extend the opportunity for supported living to all people with intellectual disabilities who seek supported living as part of their preferred lifestyle. The role of the ASL is to broker the progression of supported living based on the collective membership of committed provider organisations, and other interested groups or individuals.

The objectives of the ASL are:

- To provide a central source of support, information and knowledge-sharing among all participating members
- To address the key barriers affecting the development of supported living as they are seen by members
- To lead on the development of best practice as it relates to supported living
- To advocate for supported living as an accessible lifestyle option for people, irrespective of how much support they need to live their daily lives
- To influence the development of national policy through dialogue with government and its agents for change

The ASL represents the views of its members to government and other agencies, at a national level. The ASL is a member of the Department of Health's Intellectual Disability Task Force and the joint Healthcare Commission/Commission for Social Care Inspection's Intellectual Disability Improvement Board. The ASL, on behalf of members, has opened dialogues with the Office of the Deputy Prime Minister (Supporting People), and the Valuing People Support Team. Each year the ASL holds a national conference and other member consultative events. In partnership with the Valuing People Support Team the ASL commissioned Paradigm to revise the REACH standards. REACH 2 defines supported living for people with intellectual disabilities and is an extremely useful tool to help provider organisations ensure compliance with Domiciliary Care Standards and Supporting People.

Any organisation providing supported living for people with intellectual disabilities that aspires to meet the REACH 2 standards may join the ASL.

The current member organisations of the ASL support over 14 000 people with intellectual disabilities with combined annual budgets of over £500 million:

Benefits of membership of the ASL include:

- Membership of the only national network dedicated to promoting supported living for adults with intellectual disabilities
- A free place at the ASL's annual conference and additional discounted places
- An opportunity to shape the development of supported living at a national level
- An opportunity to express your views on issues related to supported living directly to the government and its agencies
- Copies of REACH 2 at the ASL member's rate of £20
- A range of networking opportunities at regular organised ASL events

Getting equal housing

CONCLUSION

It took 30 years to close long-stay hospitals for people with intellectual disabilities. This will remain a lasting testimony to how ineffectual official policy was in getting rid of the most appalling accommodation options to be created for people with intellectual disabilities since the proliferation of Workhouses began resulting from the 1834 Poor Law Amendment Act. Housing options for people with intellectual disabilities remain limited and there are few examples of people with intellectual disabilities 'Getting Equal Housing'. While 'Official' policy continues to fail people with intellectual disabilities it is 'Unofficial Policy' and innovation that has largely been responsible for achieving beneficial change (Duffy 1996, Rose 1993).

The case studies cited in this chapter all show how people with intellectual disabilities can be supported to 'Get Equal Housing'. The Housing Options case study 'Rebecca's story' was first published as long ago as 1996, Progress Care Housing Association have so far provided 1700 tenancies for people with intellectual disabilities and mental health problems, while Advance Housing and Support has already helped hundreds of people with intellectual disabilities to own their own homes. 'in Control' is demonstrating time and time again how self-directed support can achieve citizenship where services often fail. These innovative organisations and approaches have demonstrated just what can be achieved and these approaches are beginning to be more widely promoted through the Association for Supported Living. Others need to follow these examples. There can no longer be any excuse for the continuation of the dire situation that so many people with intellectual disabilities find themselves in, highlighted in the National Survey (Emerson et al 2005) and reported on in the introduction to this chapter, in relation to 'Getting Equal Housing'.

ACKNOWLEDGEMENTS

Maurice Harker, Housing Options, Simon Duffy, 'in Control', Lynda Mason, Progress Care Housing Association and Graeme Jackson, Advance Housing all provided information and case studies to inform this chapter.

REFERENCES

Department of Health 2001 Valuing People: a new strategy for learning disability for the 21st century. HMSO, London.

Duffy S 1996 Unlocking the imagination. Choice Press, London.

Emerson E, Malam S, Davies I, Spencer K 2005 Adults with learning difficulties in England 2003/04. Health and Social Care Information Centre, Government Statistical Service.

Harker M 2003 Housing needs and supply in England – learning disabilities background paper originally prepared for the Valuing People Support Team.

King N 1996 Ownership options. National Housing Federation.

Poll C, Duffy S, Hatton C et al 2006 A report on 'in Control's first phase. 'in Control' Publications.

Rose S J 1993 Social policy: a perspective on service developments and inter-agency working. In: Brigdon P, Todd M (eds) Concepts in community care for people with a learning difficulty. Macmillan Publishing, Basingstoke.

BIBLIOGRAPHY

Duffy S 2003 Keys to citizenship: a guide to getting good support for people with intellectual disabilities. Paradigm, Birkenhead.

CONTACT DETAILS

Housing Options
Maurice Harker
Director, Housing Options
Stanlaw House
Sutton Lane
Sutton
Witney
Oxfordshire
OX29 5RY
enquiries@housingoptions.org.uk
Tel: 0845 4561497
www.housingoptions.org.uk

'in Control'
Simon Duffy
National Director
Tel: 07973 715983
simon.duffy@in-control.org.uk

Progress Care Housing Association
Lynda Mason
Projects Manager
Progress Care Housing Association
Sumner House, 21 King Street
Leyland, Lancashire
PR25 2LW
lmason@progressgroup.org.uk
Tel: 01772 450894

Advance Housing and Support
Graeme Jackson
Head of Home Ownership
Advance Housing and Support
2 Witan Way
Witney
Oxfordshire
OX28 6FH
Graeme.jackson@advanceuk.org
Tel: 01993 772885

Association for Supported Living
Di Denham
ASL Administrator
c/o Advance Housing and Support
2 Witan Way
Witney
Oxfordshire
OX8 6FH
diane.denham@advanccuk.org
Tel: 01993 772 885

Ethnicity and intellectual disability

Raghu Raghavan

Ethnicity is a key theme in our world today. All human beings have an ethnic identity and it does not relate to just people from different nationalities, cultures or religions. The focus of this chapter is on people with intellectual disabilities from Black and Minority Ethnic (BME) communities as they face inequalities, discrimination and marginalisation. This chapter will highlight some of the key issues and themes in health and social care of people with intellectual disabilities from minority ethnic communities. These include:

- Definitions of ethnicity, culture and race
- Prevalence of learning disability in minority ethnic communities
- Religion and belief systems and the perception of intellectual disability

- Children and young people perspectives
- Family carer perspectives
- Cultural sensitivity, cultural reciprocity and cultural competence

The user and carer perspective will be presented through the use of case studies which are drawn from a number of commissioned research studies.

INTRODUCTION

The UK population is becoming gradually more diverse and complex in terms of ethnicity, culture, language and religion. According to the 2001 census, nearly 92% of the UK population are White and about 7. 9% of people are from different ethnic groups, which consist of about 4.6 million people (www. statistics.gov.uk/). The census data show that among the population of various ethnic groups, Indians are the largest, followed by Pakistanis, those of mixed ethnic backgrounds, Black Caribbeans, Black Africans and Bangladeshis. The 2001 census also collected information on ethnicity and religion. Majority of the White population are considered to be Christians and there are a number of other religious groups. Among these groups the Pakistani Muslims were the largest, followed by Indian Hindus, Indian Sikhs, Bangladeshi Muslims and White Jews.

The *Valuing People* White Paper (Department of Health 2001) outlines the Government's strategy for improving the lives of people with an intellectual disability and their families. The agenda is based on the recognition of their rights as citizens to be socially included, have choice in their daily lives and to have opportunities to achieve independence. The *Valuing People* White

Paper (Department of Health 2001:2) states that many people from minority communities are even more excluded than White people with intellectual disabilities and that 'the needs of people from minority ethnic communities are often overlooked'. *Valuing People* calls for an improvement of services so that they not only meet the needs of all people but value them as citizens.

It is well recognised that people with an intellectual disability from Black and Minority Ethnic (BME) groups are under-represented in services compared to their White counterparts (Nazroo 1997). They may experience even further isolation, as many of these people face greater inequalities in relation to race, disability and gender and exclusion in employment, education and health (Mir et al 2001). The nature of experiences such as discrimination and social exclusion of people from BME communities will make a negative impact on their health, well being and the social networks.

Often the terminology used by services and the general public about people from different cultural/religious groups is 'ethnic minority'. This may be very insulting to those described, indicating that only 'minorities' have an ethnicity (Ratcliffe 2004). We all belong to an ethnic group, and it is important to emphasise the ethnic majority. In this chapter the preferred term 'minority ethnic community or groups' is used. In this context it is important to explore the related terms used widely such as culture, race, ethnicity and cultural diversity prior to examining the issues of people with intellectual disabilities from minority ethnic communities.

WHAT IS CULTURE?

Historically, the word 'culture' has been used to describe many aspects of social life. Hellman (2001) describes culture as a set of guidelines (both implicit and explicit) that individuals inherit as members of a particular society, which informs them how to view the world, how to experience it emotionally, and how to behave in it in relation to other people, to supernatural forces and Gods, and to the natural environment.

Cultural background has a significant influence on many aspects of people's lives which include their beliefs, behaviour, perceptions, emotions, language, religion, rituals, family structure, diet, dress, body image, concepts of space and time, and attitudes to illness and pain and other forms of misfortune (Hellman 2001).

ETHNICITY

Ethnicity is a common term used in health and social sciences and the definitions include references to place of origin, or ancestry, skin colour, cultural heritage, religion and language. Ethnicity is defined as the group a person belongs to as a result of certain shared characteristics including ancestral and geographical origins, social and cultural traditions, religion and languages (Mackintosh et al 1998).

It is important to understand that we all belong to an ethnic group even though the term 'ethnic' is often incorrectly used to refer only to individuals from Black and minority backgrounds.

RACE

The term 'race' originated in relation to assumed differences on biological grounds with members of a particular racial group sharing certain distinguishing physical characteristics such as bone structure and skin colour (Giger & Davidhizar 1999). The expansion of the knowledge base about biological variations through population and genetic studies shows that there is little genetic difference between the various racial groups and hence the term race has been discredited. The Parekh Report (Runnymede Trust 2000) argues that race is a social and political construct, and not a biological or genetic fact.

CULTURAL DIVERSITY

Cultural diversity encompasses issues of perceived and real differences with respect to age, gender, ethnicity, disability, religion, lifestyles, family and kinship, dietary preferences, traditional dress, language or dialects spoken, sexual orientation, educational and occupational status, and other factors (Purnell & Paulanka 1998). In valuing diversity and the awareness of diversity, an understanding of values, beliefs, behaviours and orientations are essential.

PREVALENCE

The World Health Organization (WHO) estimates the prevalence of intellectual disability to be between 1% and 3%. Reports on the prevalence of intellectual disabilities across many countries range from 2% to 8% depending on the definition and the classification systems used (Roeleveld et al 1997). We are unable to estimate the prevalence of intellectual disabilities in all the ethnic groups in the UK due to the lack of prevalence studies in specific communities. It is reported that severe intellectual disability was three times more prevalent in South Asian (comprising Indian, Pakistani and Bangladeshi nationalities) children and young adults than in age matched peers in other ethnic groups (Emerson et al 1997). This study highlights that between the age of 5 and 34 years the prevalence of intellectual disabilities is approximately three times higher among the Asian community in comparison to the non-Asian community. This study also suggests a link between socio-economic deprivation and intellectual disabilities, which has also been emphasised in earlier research (Mclaren & Bryson 1987) that highlights the link between poverty, and rates of mild intellectual disabilities. Many studies reveal a strong link between socio-economic factors such as lack of nutrition, poor housing conditions, poor child rearing practices and high prevalence of mild intellectual disabilities (Baumeister et al 1993, Mink 1997).The prevalence of intellectual disabilities in other ethnic groups in the UK is not known.

The high prevalence of intellectual disabilities in the South Asian community is heavily contested. For example, a study conducted in Leicestershire (McGrowther et al 2002) found that the South Asian and White populations have a similar prevalence of intellectual disabilities and related psychological morbidity. This is based on the prevalence of intellectual disabilities in adults in Leicestershire which is 3.20 per 1000 in South Asians and 3.62 per 1000 Whites. Among adults with intellectual disabilities, South Asians in

Leicestershire have similar prevalence and psychological morbidity to Whites. However, the use of psychiatric services, residential and respite care services was lower by people from the South Asian community. A point to note here in comparison with the Emerson et al (1997) study is the ethnicity of the participants. Even though both are from South Asian communities, Emerson et al focused on Pakistani and Bangladeshi communities from socially deprived areas while McGrowther looked at the Indian community from privileged backgrounds.

In many South Asian cultures, first cousin marriages or consanguinity is suggested as a cause for poorer birth outcomes in South Asian communities. It is suggested that professionals often use the consanguinity to shift the blame for disability to parents and reinforce negative stereotypes of other cultures and traditions (Ahmad 1996a). However, this practice alone should not be singled out as the main causative factor, and other factors such as access to and use of antenatal health care, lack of awareness and use of genetic screening to identify the risk factors, and the problems associated with communication as a result of language barriers are significant risk factors for higher prevalence of intellectual disabilities in the South Asian community. For example, the higher prevalence has been linked to high levels of maternal and social deprivation combined with factors such as inequality in health care (Emerson et al 1997).

RELIGIOUS BELIEFS

Religious beliefs of the family play a major role in accepting the birth of a disabled child, in managing stress and exploring ways of adapting to life with a disabled child. For example, family carers of young people with intellectual disabilities in Bradford were of the opinion that the professionals and service providers often overlook the religious and cultural needs of the young person (Raghavan et al 2005). This is well captured in a statement from a Pakistani Muslim family, who said 'We've left it to Allah... we can't do anything else'.

This is also confirmed by other studies in the UK. Bywaters et al (2003) in their study of attitudes towards disability amongst Pakistani and Bangladeshi children in the UK, found that religious beliefs have a central role in the lives of parents from this community in understanding disability. Religious beliefs may help parents to cope with their own feelings and stigma. The authors argue the importance of religious or spiritual beliefs of the family and the need for health and social care professionals to be sensitive to the family's belief system while providing advice or planning services.

In examining the religious beliefs of the South Asian population, it is vital to understand the main religions practised in South Asia. These consist of Hinduism, Islam, Buddhism and Sikhism. It is reported that many Muslims accept disability as 'God's will' while Hindu and Sikh female carers' attitudes towards disability are based on the notion of Karma (Katbamna et al 2000). In examining the Hindu belief system, a two-year ethnographic study by (Gabel 2004) investigated cultural beliefs about disability among the South Asian Indian immigrants living in the mid-Western United States. This study sheds light on Hindu religious beliefs and intellectual disabilities. A key belief system is that disability is God's gift given as a result of actions (*Karma*) of past life, reflecting the Hindu belief of reincarnation or rebirth. The participants believed that intellectual disability in the family was a sign that the person labelled with intellectual disabilities or someone in the person's family had lessons from a previous life (Karma) that must be learned in the present life and they believed that having intellectual disabilities or having a loved one with intellectual disabilities would provide opportunities to learn those lessons. This study highlights the Hindu belief that one must suffer through the disability without complaint. In this context, suffering is not a negative connotation but a learning opportunity, which could provide a chance to learn lessons that could release them from rebirth as release from the cycle of birth and death is the goal of Hindu life. It is important to note the belief here – *suffering is an opportunity to willingly fulfil one's duties in life and one must do this without complaining*. This belief has major implications in terms of service access and uptake from families following the Hindu religion.

Many family carers from South Asian communities also consult religious healers in relation to their children with intellectual disabilities. In the Bradford study on young people with intellectual disabilities and mental health problems (Raghavan et al 2005) many families consulted religious or traditional healers, in the hope that they would make their child 'better'.

'Yeah, we have (used religious/traditional healers) abroad because people said somebody might have done black magic on her...so we went abroad last year. When she was there, she found it difficult because of the different people and surroundings...they thought it was to do with black magic...so they got a religious man to do things...it didn't work.'

A Pakistani family carer

Many Pakistani and Bangladeshi people felt that religion was very important in the way they led their lives (Modood & Berthoud 1997). Cinnirella & Loewenthal (1999) in their study examined religious and ethnic group influences on beliefs about mental illness and reported that faith and prayer were effective in treating mental illness and more preferred than going to see a 'holy person'. It should be noted that even though members of the South Asian community make more contact with religious healers, this does not mean that they are less likely to contact medical professionals and the participants in this study looked to both as a means of getting the help they needed (Fatimilehin & Nadirshaw 1994).

Religious beliefs have been explored in other minority ethnic groups in other countries. Skinner et al (2001) interviewed 250 parents of Mexican and Puerto Rican origin living in the United States, who had young children with developmental delays, to provide a comprehensive view of the role of religious beliefs and practices in their lives. This highlights that religious beliefs and practices provided instrumental and socio-emotional support, but faith was clearly viewed as providing more support than institutionalised religion. The findings also indicate that religion, as a system of beliefs or an interpretative framework, provided the majority of parents with a way to understand what disability meant for them, their families and relationship to God. A key factor emerging from this study is the belief system that a disabled child as part of God's plan gave parents more faith and strength and to act in the interest of their child and family, which is contrary to the fatalism. Clearly the findings from this study indicate the role of belief systems in fostering more positive interpretations and personal transformations around disability.

CHILDREN AND YOUNG PEOPLE WITH LEARNING DISABILITIES

School leavers with intellectual disabilities often face difficulties in making a smooth transition from school to college, employment or, more broadly, adult life. The transition phase is traumatic for the young person with intellectual disabilities and their families from all cultures. All young people are required to have a transition plan by the age of 14 with the young person, their family carers and all the service agencies concerned. The aim of the transition process is to ensure a smooth transition from children's services to adult services, to minimise anxieties produced by this change and to provide quality services for all these young people (Stappleton 2000). However, in practice many young people from BME communities and their parents are not aware of a transition plan (Hatton et al 2002).

Many young people from minority ethnic communities often face exclusion and isolation resulting in *'double disadvantage'* or *'triple jeopardy'* (Butt & Mirza 1996). It is expected that between the years 1991 and 2021 the number of White people with intellectual disabilities will rise by 3% while the number of non-White will rise by 70% (Emerson et al 2001). Despite this population projection, school leavers with intellectual disabilities from a South Asian background are often under-represented in formal services although the families report a great need for formal support (Hatton et al 1998, Mir et al 2001). Minority ethnic groups also experience social and material disadvantages and face barriers in their access to statutory support services in many areas of need (Chamba et al 1999). These young people experience even further isolation, as many face greater inequalities and exclusion in employment, education, health, income and benefits (Mir et al 2001).

Case study 13.1

Bushra is an 18-year-old British Pakistani who has cerebral palsy. She lives with her parents and sister. She has two other sisters, one who visits often and the other lives in another city. She has two friends at school and is also very close to her teacher. She also considers her sisters to be her friends. She does not see her friends out of school. She goes to her Mum and sisters when she needs help. They take her shopping, which she enjoys. During the holidays she visits family with her parents. She also likes to listen to music and watches videos. She is currently going to a mainstream school but will be leaving at the end of the term. At the moment she does computing and maths in school. She has been bowling with the school, which she enjoys.

She will be starting college soon. She is worried as she doesn't know if she will have 'nice' friends there. She will miss her friends and teachers. She feels sad about leaving school. She does not know what she will do after she leaves college, but thinks she will feel sad. She said 'I feel worried, don't like leaving school…nice teachers and friends'. She does not know what she wants to do in the future. She would still like to live with her parents when she is older.

The above story highlights the plight of many young people with intellectual disabilities in the transition phase. Many young people from minority ethnic communities tend to rely on their teachers and small groups of peers at school as friends, as they do not have other opportunities to make or expand their networks of friends. So, naturally they may feel lost at the stage of transition as result of losing their 'only group' of friends and face a world of uncertainties. What is important here is that many young people with intellectual disabilities from minority ethnic communities experience lack of friendship and social networks when they leave school or college. This will create a negative impact for many youngsters from minority ethnic communities in terms of perceiving their social world and their identity in society.

Many young people from BME communities have little opportunity to partake in peer support groups or advocacy groups. For example in a study by Bignall et al (2002) young people from Asian, Caribbean and African backgrounds were recruited to participate in peer support groups. The young people stated that participation in these groups allowed them greater opportunities to explore their ethnicity and to meet and be with young people similar to themselves. Attending a peer support group was important in the lives of these disabled young BME people. Participation in the groups allowed the young people to gain emotional support, make friends, learn new skills, and to enjoy themselves. Bignall et al found that a number of factors prevented young people from attending peer support groups which included transport, access to venue and money.

Leisure opportunities and involvement in leisure activities is a key factor in facilitating the development of skills and adaptive behaviour. Involvement in leisure activities is an important aspect of most of our lives. Not only is it a valuable form of entertainment but it also provides a means to establish friendships with peers and contributes to better health and wellbeing. It has been found that young people with a learning disability tend to participate in home based activities and may often be excluded from mainstream activities (Azmi et al 1997, McConkey & McGinley 1990). Research with young people and leisure from BME communities highlights that adolescents and adults with an intellectual disability from South Asian communities were consulted about their views in relation to specific areas of their lives. It was found that 'double discrimination' led to a lack of culturally appropriate services, limited friendships and a lack of leisure activities (Azmi et al 1997). It also suggested that most young people had experiences of disability that were similar to those of their White peers, some were discriminated against because of their ethnicity and felt excluded from services because their cultural needs were not being met (Hussain et al 2002). In a recent study into the leisure opportunities for young people from a South Asian community, the young people felt that they needed to be consulted by service providers for planning the leisure services that they need (Raghavan & Pawson 2007). Indeed consultation with users is a key feature of the White Paper *Our health, Our Care Our say: a new direction for community services* (Department of Health 2006) which emphasises providing a stronger voice for users in acting as major drivers for service improvement.

Ethnicity and intellectual disability

FAMILY CARER PERSPECTIVES

The UK is a multi-cultural society which consists of diverse family and cultural patterns and these differ among ethnic groups (Nazroo 1997). The multi-cultural nature of the UK population means that there are diverse perspectives on family responsibilities where norms and beliefs about family responsibilities are not easily identifiable. What we do know about family responsibilities and obligations is based on social class and gender differences (Finch & Mason 1990). Family life is an important and integral part of Asian life but is rarely explored in the British context. There is extensive literature on family relationships and the negotiation of family obligations in the majority White community in contrast to the available literature on parenting within the minority ethnic population in the UK (Ahmad 1996b). This has not been followed up with work on Asian family life in any great depth. Another problem is that the 'South Asians' tend be categorised as one group (Ahmad 1996b) which does not take into account differences between ethnic groups which can vary enormously based on culture and religious differences.

Many South Asian families may have more than one disabled child in the family, and some of these people may have severe and complex intellectual disabilities which place the families under severe stress. The White Paper *Valuing People* (Department of Health 2001) estimates that one third of people with intellectual disabilities living in the family home are living with a carer aged 70 or over. Many of these older carers have often been caring for years with very little support from services.

A major obstacle for voluntary and statutory service providers is the lack of any relevant information about the nature and type of services required by older carers from the South Asian community. We already know that older carers from the South Asian community wish to have services that would respect their cultural and religious needs (Raghavan et al 2005). Indeed many of these older carers would wish to access the services available, if they offer culturally sensitive services. In this context, it is important to explore the nature of services required by these older carers, types of support required, and to identify best ways of providing these services.

It is widely recognised that minority ethnic groups experience social and material disadvantage when accessing statutory support services, particularly families that have a disabled child. Research has shown that overall minority ethnic families who care for a severely disabled child were even more disadvantaged than White families. Such families were likely to have lower levels of employment, particularly among mothers and fewer families were receiving disability benefits and less likely to receive higher rates of Disability Living Allowance (DLA). There are particular cultural barriers such as lack of language skills in English which can hamper access and there remains a need to have interpreting services and translated material in languages other than English. There were also higher levels of unmet need for both children and parents that need to be addressed, for example respite care or short-term breaks (Chamba et al 1999).

The *Valuing People* White Paper (Department of Health 2001) stresses the importance of hearing the voices of family carers in developing policy and its implementation at national and local levels. Recent research into the views of older carers with a son or daughter with intellectual disabilities indicates that older family carers from all ethnic groups experience difficulties. However, there are specific issues in relation to older carers from minority ethnic communities, in this case from the South Asian community in Bradford (Raghavan 2007). These include:

- Language barriers
- Anxiety about cultural appropriateness of future care of their son/ daughter after their time
- Lack of awareness of support groups or family carer networks

---

Case study 13.2

Kasim is a 22-year-old male of Pakistani origin with moderate intellectual disability. At birth he appeared physically fine and the doctors did not mention any medical abnormalities to the family. It was only when he started school that the teachers identified his intellectual disability. Kasim's main carers are his mum and dad. His father is unemployed having had to give up work to look after him on a full time basis, as his mother was finding it very difficult to manage him on her own. Kasim is unable to communicate using language. He cannot read, write, tell the time, count or deal with money. He is also unable to answer the phone, personally identify himself or go out alone. He needs someone with him at all times. He will not eat unless he is fed, usually by the mum, and needs help with getting dressed, going to the toilet, bathing, oral and nasal hygiene and shaving. Kasim takes time to respond to instructions and sometimes does not listen at all. He can be very impulsive and wanders around aimlessly from room to room, on many occasions. Kasim was showing some behaviour problems at school so his father decided to tutor him at home privately, but he was not interested in learning. He has support workers and professional help, but Kasim does not like people around him. He also has limited contact with anyone outside his family, as he gets angry and aggressive with others.

Kasim is always at home and is not accessing any help or using any of the services. His daily routine consists of eating, sleeping and watching TV. Kasim has not accessed any day services or workshops before, even though the social worker had tried to organise this for him. Kasim has been displaying psychological problems and he is receiving help from a psychiatrist. His behaviour has deteriorated and he tends to get aggressive quite frequently. He throws tantrums and things around and cries frequently.

Kasim is not using any services other than the psychiatrist for medication. His father feels he does not know whom to contact to get his son the help he needs. He feels unsupported from the professionals. Kasim's father would like him to go out and partake in leisure activities and perhaps use day centres so that he can interact with other young people and get out of the house. His father wants Kasim to learn basic skills like reading, writing and counting so that he can be a little independent. Kasim will carry on staying with his parents and they are not sure what the future holds for him and it causes them a lot of concern. His father finds it very difficult to get help, as he does not speak English. Kasim is frustrated from being stuck in the house all the time, which he takes out on the carers and the carers find it very hard to look after him.

Ethnicity and intellectual disability

The above story highlights some of the frustrations and needs of an older family carer. An important barrier to service uptake for many South Asian families is language and communication. Family carers unable to speak English face particular problems in terms of access. Interpreters or link worker schemes remain inadequate with most service users relying on their young children for interpretation (Ahmad & Jones 1998). There is a need for interpreters but their use is very patchy (Hatton et al 2002). Even when service users can speak English, poor communication between them and the professional, rather than language difficulties, may limit South Asian families' understanding of diagnosis and restrict further opportunities for discussion with the professional.

Along with language and communication problems, the biggest barrier to uptake appeared to be a lack of knowledge and awareness of services. In recent research conducted in Bradford with South Asian families (Raghavan 2005, 2007) most participants reported not knowing about particular services, or how to access them or whom to ask about services. For example, a Pakistani family carer said:

> 'Getting services is difficult, so I don't ask for help. To get that help, you have to be a very clever person, how to approach them and get info…people like us can't do that…'
>
> Raghavan 2005

Most families were not equipped with enough information about the help and support they needed. The lack of knowledge and awareness about services has also been highlighted by previous research (Emerson & Robertson 2002). Chamba et al (1999) argue that given the lack of awareness and service support reported it is not surprising that unmet needs are reported so highly in this population.

Stigma is also a key factor for many family carers from South Asian communities For example, the Bradford study on young people with intellectual disabilities and mental health needs indicates that Pakistani and Bangladeshi families were worried about what others may say, especially when communities are so close-knit and people don't want sensitive issues to be found out by others in the community. For example, a family carer said, 'Asian people worry about what others say…people worry about their reputation'. Stigma and family reputations are crucial with regards to mental illness and most South Asian people want to keep such issues concerning their family members within the family structure, with carers taking extra precautions to hide any conditions associated with mental ill health (Bashford et al 2002). It is not just the young people that are suffering from mental health concerns – carers have also expressed the emotional burden the child's disability places on them. Carers report high levels of stress. It is very important to support the emotional well-being of the carers, when considering care issues for the young people (FPLD 2002) and there appears to be a need for greater awareness and understanding of mental health across all communities, not just South Asian people (Bashford et al 2002).

There are also a number of stereotypical assumptions that have been made about South Asian communities holding different attitudes from the White population. The South Asians are often described as being a close-knit community where the main characteristic of village life is that everyone knows each other: close friends are classified as 'brothers' and 'sisters' (Khan 1979). The stereotypical view of South Asian families is that they stick together and help each other in times of need and hardship as we will see that, among some single-parent families who have a disabled child, support from outside the immediate family can be limited or even non-existent in some cases. Some service providers have been slow to acknowledge this. It is inappropriate to assume that all Pakistani and Bangladeshi parents will hold the same views (Begum 1992). There is heterogeneity of views and opinions in this community as in others. Some of these stereotypical views have been used to explain why minority ethnic families have lower uptake of services than White families, which is a way of blaming the victim and minimising the problem of institutional racism (Ahmad & Atkin 1996). Research has also demonstrated that South Asian families with a young person with intellectual disabilities receive less support from extended families than White families (Chamba et al 1999, Mir et al 2001). However the myth of the large extended family giving support has led to the view that people from minority ethnic communities do not need formal support (Atkin & Rollings 1996). There has also been a tendency to blame religious beliefs and shame of having a disabled child as reasons for low service usage (Bywaters et al 2003).

CULTURAL SENSITIVITY AND CULTURAL COMPETENCE

People with intellectual disabilities and their carers from BME communities have a lower take up of services, which may be due to language and communication difficulties, lack of awareness of services and lack of accessible information, lack of cultural sensitivity and awareness by service providers and their negative past experiences. The report by Mir et al (2001) on ethnicity and intellectual disabilities stresses the need for services to work closely with people with intellectual disabilities and their family carers from BME communities. This report recommends five key areas for development for services. These are:

- Services need to take account of the particular needs and values
- Partnerships with minority ethnic groups are needed to influence local service planning
- The role of advocacy
- Addressing the restrictive attitudes towards disability within minority communities
- Increased participation and control for people with intellectual disabilities from minority ethnic communities in service planning.

Along with the language and communication barriers and awareness of services, there other important issues that service providers and commissioners need to consider in the planning and delivery of culturally sensitive services for people from minority ethnic communities. Firstly, the services offered should be appropriate to the person with intellectual disabilities and their family. One of the primary reasons for low take up of services is the inappropriate nature of services. The types of services offered are often not appropriate to meet their needs; for example, providing a support worker without any satisfactory awareness and knowledge of intellectual disability and cultural awareness creates more stress and work for the families, rather than helping them. Secondly, some services might indicate that they treat all their users equally. A 'colour-blind' approach where the services are offered to all users poses a barrier for people from minority ethnic communities. This type of approach ignores the cultural values and belief systems of the users as it creates a negative view of services for them. People from minority ethnic communities are not seeking a specially created service for them. Instead, they wish for mainstream services to be more accommodative of their views and needs. This can be achieved by involving people with intellectual disability and their carers from minority ethnic communities in terms of planning services. 'Hearing the voice' and creating opportunities for 'visibility' of users and carers from minority ethnic communities is essential in building inclusive services that meet the needs of people in the locality.

Users and carers from all sections of the local community should be involved in engaging with their local services. Naturally, it is important to hear the voice of people from minority ethnic communities for planning and shaping the service delivery. This will require a concerted effort by commissioners and providers to identify users and carers from minority communities and to enable them to attend planning meetings. In order to attend these meetings the users and carers will require additional help and support such as the availability of an interpreter, flexibility in terms of the timing of the meeting to accommodate their cultural and religious needs, and more importantly having the willingness to engage in a dialogue with users and carers from this community without any preconceived ideas about the nature of services that they may require. One such initiative was conducted in Bradford recently in terms of planning the leisure services for young people with intellectual disabilities from the South Asian community. This involved recruiting and coaching a core group of youngsters with learning disabilities representing the heterogeneity in the South Asian community and providing opportunities for these youngsters and family carers to have a series of meetings with key service providers in the locality. This involved extensive planning and external facilitation and was funded by MENCAP (Raghavan & Pawson 2007). As a result of the meetings with users, carers and service providers, a clear plan of action for accessing leisure services was drawn up which was agreed by all parties. For services up and down the country such initiatives of joint planning will provide fruitful benefits in terms of having a reference group from minority ethnic communities for planning and shaping the services of tomorrow.

The use of a key worker has been suggested by Hatton et al (2002) and Emerson & Robertson (2002) in supporting young people and family carers from South Asian communities. The key emphasis here is for the key worker to be a person from the minority community so that they are able to communicate effectively using the appropriate language. The key worker might also help to link up the family with a range of service providers and professionals, thus helping to access the range of services. Such a service model, through the use of a liaison worker, was tested with young people with learning disabilities and mental health needs from a Pakistani and Bangladeshi community (Raghavan et al in press). This was a pilot randomised controlled trial (RCT) to evaluate the effectiveness of a liaison worker with this community to increase the access to services. Two randomised groups of young people with intellectual disabilities and mental health needs were set up, a treatment group (n = 12) and a control group (n = 14). Both groups were able to access the standard statutory and voluntary services, but the treatment group had the additional help of a liaison worker and the control group had no additional help from the liaison worker. This RCT was conducted for a period of 9 months, and the main outcome measure agreed at the start of the trial was number of contacts with services, since this best reflected the aim of the study to determine whether introduction of the specialist liaison worker could enhance access to such services. It was predicted that those allocated to the liaison worker would have more contact, greater variety of contact and more outcomes of contact with services than those in the control group. Baseline assessments were conducted with young people and their family carers at the beginning and end of the trial. The findings of this trial indicate that the liaison worker model was found to be useful by families. Families receiving input from the liaison worker had more frequent contact with more services than did families not receiving this input and had more results from such contacts. There was also some indication that family carers receiving support had a better quality of life and the young person with intellectual disabilities had fewer behavioural problems than controls. This shows that the model of a liaison worker may be effective in supporting people with intellectual disabilities and their carers from minority ethnic communities.

The *Valuing People* strategy emphasises the planning of local services to meet the needs of people with intellectual disabilities and their carers. This is to be achieved through Partnership Boards with representation from people with intellectual disabilities and carers and all service providers and agencies. *Learning Difficulties and Ethnicity: A Framework for Action Guide* (Department of Health 2004) stresses that Partnership Boards should have representation from minority ethnic communities. This framework is beneficial for Partnership Boards to examine their local population and to explore their links and representation from minority ethnic groups, support of voluntary organisations, the need to recruit and retain a workforce from minority ethnic communities and to review the policy and practice in the locality with special reference to ethnicity. It should be borne in mind that for effective inclusion of people with intellectual disabilities and their carers from all sections of the minority communities in the locality in the Partnership Board, every effort should be made to hear the diverse views of users and carers from this community and should steer clear of 'token' representation that only provides a skewed view of their needs and services.

Developing culturally sensitive services is a high priority agenda for commissioners and service providers. Malek (2004) argues that delivering culturally sensitive services requires recognition of cultural beliefs and practices at the grassroots level of service delivery and also at the strategic level of service planning. In order to do these, Malek indicates a key range of activities such as:

- A policy framework that supports a culturally sensitive response at all levels
- Data collection on minority ethnic communities generally and the number of people from minority ethnic groups attending each service
- Research into theory and practice issues necessary to develop and deliver culturally sensitive practice
- Collaboration with ethnic and other agencies to ensure that the needs of specific ethnic groups are understood and addressed
- Education for staff
- Administrative structures that support the delivery of culturally sensitive services
- Training of clinical and administrative staff to respond sensitively and competently when dealing with people from a range of cultures

It is not only cultural sensitivity that is paramount in shaping and delivering services to people from minority ethnic communities, but in addition the workforce needs to be culturally competent. Cultural competence is the development of skills by individuals and systems to live and work with, educate and serve diverse individuals and communities. It is the willingness and ability of a system to value the importance of culture in the delivery of services to all segments of the population. It is the use of a systems perspective which values differences and is responsive to diversity at all levels of an organisation, i.e. policy, governance, administrative, workforce, provider, and consumer/client. Cultural competence is developmental, community focused, family oriented, and culturally relevant. In particular, it is the attention to the needs of underserved and racial/ethnic groups, and the integration of cultural attitudes, beliefs, and practices into diagnosis and treatment, education and training, and workplace environments. It is the continuous promotion of skills, practices and interactions to ensure that services are culturally responsive and competent. Culturally competent activities include developing skills through training, using self-assessment tools, and implementing goals and objectives to ensure that governance, administrative policies and practices, and clinical skills and practices are responsive to diversity within the populations served.

CONCLUSION

People with intellectual disabilities from minority ethnic communities are likely to face exclusion and discrimination in terms of accessing and use of services. As we have seen, a number of factors such as cultural and religious beliefs, language barriers, lack of adequate knowledge and awareness of services act as barriers in accessing and using a range of services and professional help. The experiences of people with intellectual disabilities and their carers highlighted provide us with key issues to consider and to act upon as professionals and service agencies. Firstly, respecting human rights and equality, services need to take on the challenge of providing services to all sections of the community. Service commissioners should have a clear understanding of the population that they are serving and this requires having up-to-date information about the number of people from various minority ethnic communities in their geographical area. Not just having this information in the service database alone will sufficiently contribute to shaping a culturally sensitive and culturally competent service structure. This will require real effort and commitment by service agencies through consultation and active dialogue with these communities in understanding the needs of minority ethnic communities and having their involvement in service planning.

Secondly, as we have seen, many people with intellectual disabilities and their carers from minority ethnic communities may not voluntarily come forward to represent their views and opinions in terms of the kind of services they wish for and their views in making this happen in their locality. This will require active facilitation by service agencies through employment of people from minority ethnic communities and in using these people to help, support and to hear the views of people with intellectual disabilities from these communities. For making this a reality services need to formulate a clear strategy for active and continuous involvement of users from all sections of the community. The voice of family carers, especially from minority ethnic communities, should also form part of the strategy. The Learning Disability Partnership Boards have a key role in seeking and hearing the voice of users and carers from minority communities and to have their representation in their working groups which is currently lacking. This has the double advantage of enabling the users and carers and also in building trust and confidence for sustained involvement with these communities.

And finally, the workforce needs to be culturally sensitive and competent to deliver services that meet the needs of people from all sections of the community. Building culturally sensitive services has been a slogan for some years in the policy directives from the UK government. But the impact of these directives on commissioners and service providers in acting to build a culturally sensitive and culturally competent workforce is not very clear. We have limited awareness of the processes and mechanisms used by services in building a culturally competent workforce. This theme warrents closer examination in terms of the initiatives used by services and its impact on service delivery and user satisfaction through applied research. Just paying lip service for cultural competency alone will not have an impact in shaping the future services. But what will help is having the willingness and motivation by services in creating a culturally competent workforce through adequate training, monitoring and feedback. Such an initiative will help the workforce to understand the nature of issues affecting the diverse communities and the ways of helpful positioning by professionals and other service personnel. We live in an age where users have active involvement in shaping the nature of service they receive and in making this a reality it is vital that the workforce is able to understand and respond to their needs and wishes in a responsible manner that respects the cultural and belief systems of the population.

REFERENCES

Ahmad W 1996a Consanguinity and related demons: science and racism in the debate on consanguinity and birth outcomes. In: South N, Samson C (eds) The social construction of social policy. Macmillan, Basingstoke.

Ahmad W 1996b The trouble with culture. In: Kelleher D, Hillier S (eds) Researching cultural differences in health. Routledge, London.

Ahmad W, Jones L 1998 Ethnicity, health and health care in the UK. In: Peterson A (ed) Health matters. Allen and Unwin, London.

Ahmad W I U, Atkin K 1996 Race and community care. Open University Press, Buckingham.

Atkin K, Rollings J 1996 Looking after their own? Family care-giving among Asian and Afro-Caribbean communities. In: Ahmad W, Atkin K (eds) Race and community care. Open University Press, Buckingham.

Azmi S, Emerson E, Caine A, Hatton C 1997 Improving services for Asian people with learning disabilities and their families. Hester Adrian Research Centre, The University of Manchester.

Bashford J, Kaur J, Winters M, Williams R, Patel K 2002 What are the mental health needs of Bradford's Pakistani Muslim children and young people and how can they be addressed? University of Central Lancashire, Preston.

Baumeister A A, Kupstas F D, Woodley-Zanthos P 1993 The new morbidity: Recommendations for action and an updated guide to state planning for the prevention of mental retardation and related disabilities associated with socio-economic conditions. US Department of Health and Human Services, Washington DC.

Begum N 1992 Something to be proud of. Waltham Forest Race Relations Unit, London.

Bignall T, Butt J, Pagarani D 2002 Something to do: The development of peer support groups for young black and minority ethnic disabled people. Joseph Rowntree Foundation, York.

Butt J, Mirza K 1996 Social care and black communities. Race Equality Unit, London.

Bywaters P, Ali Z, Fazil Q, Wallace LM, Singh G 2003 Attitudes towards disability amongst Pakistani and Bangladeshi parents of disabled children in the UK: considerations for service providers and the disability movement. Health and Social Care in the Community 11(6):502-509.

Chamba R, Ahmad W, Hirst M et al 1990 On the edge: minority ethnic families caring for a severely disabled child. Policy Press, Bristol.

Cinnirella M, Loewenthal K 1999 Religious and ethnic group influences on beliefs about mental illness: a qualitative interview study. British Journal of Medical Psychology 72(4):505-524.

Department of Health 2001 Valuing People: a strategy for people with learning disabilities for the 21st century. The Stationery Office, London.

Department of Health 2004 Learning difficulties and ethnicity: a framework for action guide. Department of Health, London.

Department of Health 2006 Our health, our care our say: a new direction for community services. The Stationery Office, London.

Emerson E, Robertson J 2002 Future demand for services for young people with learning disabilities from South Asian and Black communities in Birmingham. Institute of Health Research, Lancaster University.

Emerson E, Azmi S, Hatton C 1997 Is there an increased prevalence of severe learning disabilities among British Asians? Ethnicity and Health 2:317-321.

Emerson E, Hatton C, Felce D, Murphy G 2001 Learning disabilities: the fundamental facts. The Foundation for People with Learning Disabilities, London.

Fatimilehin I, Nadirshaw Z 1994 A cross-cultural study of parental attitudes and beliefs about learning disability (mental handicap). Mental Handicap Research 7(3):202-226.

Finch J, Mason J 1990 Gender, employment and responsibilities to kin. Work, Employment & Society 4(3):349-367.

FPLD 2002 Count us in: the report of the committee of enquiry into meeting the mental health needs of young people with learning disabilities. Foundation for People with Learning Disabilities, London.

Gabel S 2004 South Asian Indian cultural orientations toward mental retardation. Mental Retardation 42:12-25.

Giger J N, Davidhizar R E 1999 Transcultural nursing: Assessment and Intervention, 3rd edn. Mosby, St Louis.

Hatton C, Azmi S, Caine A, Emerson E 1998 Informal carers of adolescents and adults with learning disabilities from South Asian communities. British Journal of Social Work 28:821-837.

Hatton C, Akram Y, Shah R et al 2002 Supporting South Asian families with a child with severe disabilities: A report to the Department of Health. Lancaster University, Institute for Health Research.

Hellman C G 2001 Culture, health and illness, 4th edn. Butterworth Heineman, Oxford.

Hussain Y, Atkin C, Ahmed W 2002 South Asian disabled young people and their families. Policy Press, Joseph Rowntree Foundation.

Katbamna S, Bhakta P, Parker G 2000 Perceptions of disability and care-giving relationships in South Asian communities. In: Ahmad W (ed) Ethnicity, disability and chronic illness. Open University Press, Buckingham.

Khan V 1979 Minority families in Britain: support and stress. Macmillan, London.

Mackintosh J, Bhopal R, Unwin N, Ahmad N 1998 Step by step guide to epidemiological health needs assessment for minority ethnic groups. University of Newcastle, Newcastle.

Malek M 2004 Meeting the needs of minority ethnic groups in the UK. In: Malek M, Joughin C (eds) Mental Health services for Minority Ethnic Children and Adolescents. Jessica Kingsley, London.

McConkey R, McGinley P 1990 Innovations in leisure and recreation for persons with a mental handicap. Brothers of Charity Services, Chorley.

McGrowther C W, Bhaumik S, Thorp C F et al 2002 Prevalence, morbidity and service need among South Asian and white adults with intellectual disability in Leicestershire, UK. Journal of Intellectual Disability Research 46:299-309.

McLaren J, Bryson S E 1987 Review of recent epidemiological studies of mental retardation: prevalence, associated disorders, and aetiology. American Journal of Mental Retardation 92:243-254.

Mink I T 1997 Studying culturally diverse families of children with mental retardation. International Review of Research in Mental Retardation 20:75-98.

Mir G, Nocon A, Ahmad W, Jones L 2001 Learning Difficulties and Ethnicity. Department of Health, London.

Modood T, Berthoud R 1997 Ethnic minorities in Britain: diversity and disadvantage. Policy Studies Institute, London.

Nazroo J Y 1997 The health of Britain's ethnic minorities: Findings from a National Survey. Policy Studies Institute, London.

Purnell L D, Paulanka B J 1998 Transcultural health care: a culturally competent approach. F A Davis, Philadelphia.

Raghavan R, Waseem F, Small N, Newell R 2005 Supporting young people with learning disabilities and mental health needs from a minority ethnic community. Making us count: identifying and improving mental health support for young people with learning disabilities. Foundation for People with Learning Disabilities, London.

Raghavan R 2007 The issues affecting older family carers (50+) of people with a learning disability within the Bradford district with special reference to ethnicity. Report to Mencap, Bradford.

Raghavan R, Pawson N 2007 The Aawaaz Project: leisure and young people with learning disabilities from South Asian communities. Mencap, London.

Raghavan R, Waseem F, Newell R, Small N A Randomised controlled trial of liaison worker model for young people with learning disabilities and mental health needs. Journal of Applied Research in Intellectual Disabilities (in press).

Ratcliffe P 2004 Race, ethnicity and difference: imagining the inclusive society. Open University Press, Maidenhead.

Roeleveld H, Zielhuis GA, Gabreels F 1997 The prevalence of mental retardation: a critical review of recent literature. Developments in Medical Child Neurology 39:125-132.

Runnymede Trust 2000 The future of multi-ethnic Britain. The Parekh Report. Profile Books, London.

Skinner D G, Correa V, Skinner M, Bailey D B Jr 2001 Role of religion in the lives of Latino families of young children with developmental delays. American Journal on Mental Retardation 106:297-313.

Stappleton 2000 Transitions – need it be traumatic? Bulletin 12(3):7-11.

LIVERPOOL JOHN MOORES UNIVERSITY
LEARNING SERVICES

Service users' involvement in higher education

John Lahiff

Recently, I was somewhat taken aback by a conversation I had with an academic colleague in which we talked about the involvement of users of various health and social care services in the development and provision of Higher Education (HE). I was proudly describing the roles that numerous people with intellectual disabilities had played in the development and implementation of a new intellectual disability nursing curriculum at Coventry and Worcester Universities. My colleague, who doesn't work in the intellectual disability field, appeared to resent the notion of user involvement in HE – at least that was the impression I was left with. Similar conversations have no doubt occurred in various HE organisations around the country, and service user involvement in HE is therefore at something of a crossroads. From service users themselves through to government policy, user involvement is widely advocated and encouraged. However, in HE, like elsewhere, substantial resistance remains.

This chapter seeks to explore some of the reasons for this, including some of the structural and philosophical issues, concerns and challenges underlying current service user involvement debates. User involvement has many perceived benefits, but it is essential, and the purpose of this chapter, that these are considered critically, not least if real and meaningful service user involvement and influence are to be achieved.

INTRODUCTION

Higher education (HE) has two main areas of focus – education and research, in this instance, health & social care education and research. In the intellectual disability field in particular, the involvement of service users in HE has on the one hand become much more widely advocated, and yet on the other, is increasingly criticised for a number of reasons. Perhaps more accurately, what is most contentious is the level of *influence*, rather than the *involvement*, of service users in HE activities. For example, people with an intellectual disability have always played a role in HE education and research (Mittler 1979). However, this role has traditionally been one of subservience or at least one of passivity. In other words it was typically the academic or researcher who established, controlled and ultimately disseminated knowledge from an academic, as opposed to the world view from the service user. It is widely acknowledged that during the past three decades, 'monumental strides' have taken place in the learning disability field (see for example,

Williams 2005), and it might therefore be expected that HE, with its reputation for innovation and cutting edge development, would be a key ally in the vanguard of the service user involvement movement. In some respects it is, examples of which will be discussed below. However, and perhaps more surprisingly, the academic community is divided as to the value, nature and purpose of service user involvement in academic study and research, and not always for antithetical reasons. Not all service users or academics are convinced that current constructions of service user involvement in HE are either appropriate or effective, nor fundamentally in the interests of service users themselves.

Superficially at least, service user involvement in HE activity is a widely accepted principle within the academic community.

THE BEGINNINGS OF SERVICE USER INVOLVEMENT IN HIGHER EDUCATION

Approximately 30 years ago Peter Mittler, in his discussion of mental handicap (*sic*) staff training and the development of training courses, suggested that those with responsibility for education should liaise with relevant stakeholders and suggested somewhat tentatively, that:

> 'parents of handicapped people, and on occasion handicapped people themselves, are joining in with professional staff to take part in discussions of new developments and consider ways in which local services and collaboration can be improved in the light of our growing knowledge of good practice and advances in knowledge and research.'
>
> Mittler 1979:207

It is interesting to note that people with an intellectual disability were, even then, beginning to take a more active role, albeit a limited one. Mittler's observation of 'occasional' service user and carer involvement would clearly suggest that these were the exception rather than the rule with no evidence to suggest that this was more widely encouraged at the time, let alone particularly well developed or established. However, positive developments were clearly taking place, albeit in a similarly embryonic fashion, for example in the research arena. Walmsley & Johnson (2003) refer to the late 1980s as the time when methodologies that sought to include and involve people with an intellectual disability in research began to emerge. One reason for this, according to Barnes et al (1999), was disenchantment with traditional disability research and, by implication, HE, that can be traced back to the 1960s. This was in no small part the result of longstanding and sometimes virulent criticism of the traditional approach to research and hierarchies of knowledge, for example by Oliver (1992) who described them as a 'rip-off', not least because they were seen to actually undermine oppressed groups at the expense of social and political imperatives. In many contemporary HE establishments service user involvement and influence is well developed with some extremely innovative and influential examples of service user academic study and research. However, the observations by Oliver (1992) appear to lie at the heart of the tensions and criticisms of contemporary provision.

DRIVERS FOR SERVICE USER INVOLVEMENT

Currently there is a widespread expectation that people with an intellectual disability will not only be involved in, but more importantly, will meaningfully influence, intellectual disability focused education and research. Many commentators point to current and past (UK) central government policy drivers for consumer involvement, beginning with the NHS and Community Care Act (1990) as key to the development of service user involvement in both research (see for example Smith et al 2008) and education and training (Repper & Breeze 2007). The national agenda, as elaborated in 'Valuing People' (Department of Health 2001a) and 'Nothing about us without us' (Department of Health 2001b) encouraging, if not obliging health and social care agencies as well as universities to work more closely in 'partnership' with people with an intellectual disability.

Likewise, national bodies involved in the funding, quality assurance, regulation, or support of HE teaching such as the Higher Education Funding Council for England (HEFCE 2007), the Quality Assurance Agency for Higher Education (QAA 2007), and Social Care Institute for Excellence (SCIE) (see for example Branfield et al 2007) are keen to ensure that partnership working and service user involvement are developed and furthermore clearly evidenced in academic activities. This is reiterated by professional regulatory bodies, who for more than a decade have equally advocated such involvement (i.e. General Medical Council 1993, CCETSW 1994, ENB 1996). Underpinning all of these is the longstanding desire and demand from the disability movement to be given a central role in determining the academic and research agenda (see for example Oliver 1992).

SERVICE USER INVOLVEMENT: IN WHOSE INTEREST IS IT ANYWAY?

'If the University wants to work in partnership with people who have learning disabilities...they'll have to look at what's best for the University, what are the students going to get out of it and what are people with learning difficulties going to get out of it?'

Boxall et al 2004:103

This quote, from a man who describes himself as an intellectual disability adult, is remarkable in at least two respects. Firstly, it reflects the tremendous inroads into the academic world made by people with an intellectual disability and in a relatively short period of time. It is unlikely that even the most ambitious or optimistic commentator three decades ago would have predicted that a person with an intellectual disability would have their views recorded and published in a well respected academic journal, let alone their views about HE and universities in particular. Secondly, Docherty offers a balanced and insightful summary of some of the complexities in the development of service user involvement in HE, not least in terms of the potentially competing interests of the parties concerned. It also leads to the question that, given the apparently longstanding and broad national and increasingly international consensus for user involvement in HE, why it is that this is not already deeply embedded in academic study and research?

One common criticism as to why change may not be happening to the extent expected is what Carr (2004) describes as 'lack of organisational responsiveness'. In other words, HE organisations, as perhaps with health and social care services, can't or won't respond sufficiently to the above social, political, financial or regulatory, or indeed user group, pressures. At least two explanations are emerging as to why this might be the case. Both positions are cognisant of the socio-political agenda and both seek to increase and enhance the influence of service users. What is in dispute, however, is the underlying purpose and therefore ultimate value of service user involvement within the current climate. Cowden & Singh (2007) for example, echoing Oliver's 'rip-off' criticism mentioned earlier, question the motivation in some quarters for the support of service user involvement in that there may be other surreptitious motives that run contrary to the wider and more fundamental interests of service users. In other words, it is argued that current user involvement constructions potentially support a covert strategy that deflects the spotlight away from a disabling society and in fact utilises user involvement to sustain the status quo, through what Carr (2004, 2007) refers to as a 'technology of legitimation'. Consequently, the push for user involvement might, unless closely monitored, turn out in reality to be a vehicle for surreptitiously reinforcing inappropriate systems and structures that are already determined to be exclusionary and oppressive. In historical terms this might be akin to inviting service users on to the management board of a large institution. In such a scenario the institution would be able to openly and honestly demonstrate and support the increased involvement and influence of service users without necessarily actually acknowledging, let alone addressing, the fundamental societal and structural deficits that the very existence of the institution reflects. As Pease (2002) points out, there is a danger in accepting a discourse that sees no need for further justification or critique, thereby opening up the possibility of a more 'subtle' form of domination.

Other commentators (Boxall et al 2004, Hanley 2005) point negatively to HE as itself a source of oppression and exclusion resulting from a defence of existing power relations, a position resonant with the views of Foucault (1980). Universities and academics traditionally pride themselves on their autonomy, which service user involvement potentially threatens and undermines because it challenges the existing power structure. Historically, people with an intellectual disability have always played an essential, but limited, passive and low status role in higher, particularly professional, education and research, namely that of being a source of data – 'the subject' or 'case'. In other words, traditionally the academic 'worth' of service users has been determined by their suitability for academic study, research, or professional practice, which in turn legitimises their exploitation. It has therefore been argued that the main challenges to service user involvement in HE lies within HE itself in that anything that challenges the power and status of 'the academy', such as user involvement and influence, will be resisted, regardless of any social, political, financial, or other pressures.

A number of barriers to user involvement within HE have been suggested, including academic and professional structures and strictures, language, and control of breadth and depth of involvement (see for example, Barnes et al 1999, Basset et al 2006, Lathlean et al 2006, Simons et al 2007). In other words, people with learning disabilities have been or are involved in HE only to the point where it benefits the academic study or research, and only as far as the power imbalance and the role of the expert or professional remains unchallenged (Manthorpe 2000). Similarly, commentators point to the continued biasing of research towards a profession centric world view (see for example Glasby & Beresford 2006, Hanson et al 2006, Kitchin 2000), continuing and in all likelihood protecting the power imbalance discussed earlier. Beresford (2007) highlights the underlying 'philosophical, moral and methodological' challenges that arise and indeed argues that service user involvement and traditional research approaches dominant in HE are incompatible. Service user involvement in research cannot be seen as neutral or 'objective' in the traditional scientific sense, but must ultimately form part of a movement for social and structural change (Walmsley & Johnson 2003). Therefore service user involvement is ultimately political in nature, and it's possible that HE is unwilling to face this for fear of offending its primary paymasters.

Other barriers can also mitigate against user involvement, as identified, for example, by Beresford et al (2006), Tyler (2006), Basset et al (2006). Some are cultural in nature, i.e. resistance from academics or the institution due to notions of 'best' knowledge or teaching being their preserve rather than that of 'outsiders'. Some are technical, in the sense that academic processes such as course development and approval can appear overly complicated, and these can be further alienating through the use of jargon. Other barriers are organisational such as physical access and payment difficulties. All the above barriers can be, and in some places have been, overcome at least where service user involvement is seen as a positive development.

From a learning perspective it would appear that service user involvement in HE has potentially a great deal to offer the student. One note of caution at this point is that there is relatively little, albeit growing, evidence currently available about the tangible impact of service user involvement, whether in relation to services (Carr 2004), or education and research (Repper & Breeze 2007). As Fisher (2002) points out there is a strong 'moral case' for user involvement but little literature in the way of benefits. That is not to say that there are no benefits, or that substantive changes have yet to take place, merely that much more investigation needs to take place in order to allow more detailed evaluation.

Of the data available, some benefits are clearly emerging for users and carers, academics and not least students. For example Simons et al (2007) identify not just positive outcomes for students, but positive developments within the academic team, largely challenging existing values and expectations. Similarly Tew et al (2004) identify a range of actual or potential benefits, and indeed go as far to suggest that user or carer led sessions may be 'the best input of the entire course', and they also note the potential cultural changes in both academic study and professional practice. Over and above this it should also be recognised that disabled people themselves have fundamentally changed our understanding of disability through the social model of disability.

SERVICE USER INVOLVEMENT AND INFLUENCE IN HIGHER EDUCATION – A CASE STUDY

The following is an example of recent and continuing service user involvement in two HE institutions (HEIs). Although briefly outlined, hopefully the reader will recognise the relationship between this scenario and the issues raised previously.

In September 2005, the first students entered the Universities of Coventry and Worcester to begin their 3 years of training to become intellectual disability nurses. The course had been approximately 2 years in the planning, involving over 100 people with intellectual disabilities and/or their carers. At that time, neither Coventry nor Worcester had been offering intellectual disability nurse training, and this was seen as an opportunity for the two universities jointly to consider the needs of service users and the structure of an appropriate course. It has been increasingly realised that the health needs of people with intellectual disabilities are poorly addressed (see for example, Signposts for Success 1998, Valuing People 2001). Service users and service providers, alongside the two HEIs sought to make local provision to meet local needs. It is worth noting that this was the first totally new intellectual disability nurse training programme for some decades, and in many respects its inception ran counter to national political and social trends. However, service users and carers clearly looked for a particular professional that would meet their particular requirements and the intellectual disability nursing programme at Coventry and Worcester was therefore born. Karl, for example, found it very frustrating that other professionals were unable to fully understand his intellectual disability and the effect that this had on his lifestyle. He saw the development of the nursing programme as a way for people to pay particular attention to this issue.

Once the programme was approved, a number of service users met several times in order to discuss their continued involvement. To date, this has included interviewing staff teaching on the programme; interviewing candidates seeking a place on the course; teaching of students on this, and other courses, including formal lectures and small groupwork; formatively assessing student communication/interviewing skills; developing visual and video materials for teaching. It was important for service users that the quality of their input was suitably high, and Laurence, for example, argued that any video material needed to be of professional standard, not just for the benefit of those video'd but also for the benefit of the students or those viewing the material. Similarly, some service users were willing to deliver lectures in a lecture hall but wished to be assured that the venue was appropriate to themselves as visiting lecturers but also for the audience, including access and availability of teaching aids.

Students have invariably commented that they have found service user led teaching sessions to be both useful and interesting. A typical comment for example from one student was that the theory around epilepsy can be somewhat dry, but when someone tells you how it affects them in their daily lives, it makes the topic much more relevant.

In addition to specific learning outcomes, there are additional benefits. For example two service users, Karl and David, delivered a talk in a traditional lecture hall setting to a large group of student nurses, following which students commented not just on the information that was delivered, but about their changed perceptions of people with intellectual disabilities. One student commented, for example, that the first time they had to speak to a group they were nearly physically sick beforehand, and was therefore extremely impressed and surprised that these two gentlemen were able to present so ably. In addition, numerous students have stated that the involvement of service users in their training will positively influence their future professional practice. As these students are yet to qualify, it will hopefully be proved an accurate prediction.

CONCLUSION

The involvement of service users in higher education activities, particularly academic study and research in health and social care related areas, has grown significantly in recent years, at least quantitatively. There are, or appear to be, potentially huge benefits to be derived by universities, students and people with intellectual difficulties. However, complete consensus has yet to be achieved as to whether or not service user involvement is actually in the long term, wider interest of users. Only through further research, evaluation and debate can this be addressed, and herein lies a particularly important, possibly extremely unpopular role for higher education. The greatest threat to the empowerment of people with an intellectual disability is a reticent and tokenistic acceptance and portrayal of user involvement. Higher education can gain in many ways from involving service users in both education and research, but such involvement must be approached appropriately.

REFERENCES

Barnes C, Mercer G, Shakespeare T 1999 Exploring disability: a sociological introduction. Polity Press, Cambridge.

Basset T, Campbell P, Anderson J 2006 Service user/survivor involvement in mental health training and education: Overcoming the barriers. Social Work Education 25(4):393-402.

Beresford P, Branfield F, Taylor J 2006 Working together for better social work education. Social Work Education 25(4):326-331.

Beresford P 2007 User involvement, research and health inequalities: developing new directions. Health and Social Care in the Community 15(4):306-312.

Boxall K, Carson I, Docherty D 2004 Room at the Academy? People with learning difficulties and higher education. Disability and Society 19(2):99-112.

Branfield F, Beresford P, Levin E 2007 Common aims: a strategy to support service user involvement in social work education. Social Care Institute for Excellence, London.

Carr S 2004 Has service user participation made a difference to social care services? Position Paper no 3. Social Care Institute for Excellence, London.

Carr S 2007 Participation, power, conflict and change: theorizing dynamics of service user participation in the social care system of England and Wales. Critical Social Policy 27(2):266-276.

CCETSW (Central Council for Education and Training in Social Work) 1994 Changing the culture: involving service users in social work education. CCESTW.

Cowden S, Singh S 2007 The 'User': Friend, foe or fetish? A critical exploration of user involvement in health and social care. Critical Social Policy 27(1):5-23.

Department of Health 2001a Valuing People: a new strategy for learning disability for the 21st century. Cm 5086. HMSO, London.

Department of Health 2001b Nothing about us without us. Department of Health, London.

ENB (English National Board for Nursing, Midwifery and Health Visiting) 1996 Learning from each other. ENB.

Fisher M 2002 The role of service users in problem formulation and technical aspects of social research. Social Work Education 21(3):305-312.

Foucault M 1980 Power/knowledge: selected writings and interviews 1972-77. Harvester Press, Brighton.

General Medical Council 1993 Tomorrow's doctors: recommendations on undergraduate medical education. GMC, London.

Glasby J, Beresford P 2006 Who knows best? Evidence-based practice and the service user contribution. Critical Social Policy 26(1):268-284.

Hanley B 2005 Research as empowerment? Report of a series of seminars organised by the Toronto group. Joseph Rowntree Trust.

Hanson E, Magnusson L, Nolan J, Nolan M 2006 Developing a model of participatory research involving researchers, practitioners, older people and their family carers: an international collaboration. Journal of Research in Nursing 11:325-342.

HEFCE (Higher Education Funding Council for England) 2007 HEFCE Strategic Plan 2006–2011: updated April 2007. HEFCE.

Kitchin R 2000 The researched opinions on research: disabled people and disability research. Disability and Society 15(1):25-47.

Lathlean J, Burgess A, Coldham T 2006 Experiences of service user and carer participation in health care education. Nurse Education Today 26:732-737.

Manthorpe J 2000 Developing carers' contributions to social work training. Social Work Education 19(1):19-27.

Mittler P 1979 People not patients: problems and policies in mental handicap. Methuen, London.

Oliver M 1992 Changing the social relations of research production. Disability Handicap & Society 7(2):101-114.

Pease B 2002 Rethinking empowerment: a postmodern reappraisal for emancipatory practice. British Journal of Social Work 32:135-147.

QAA (Quality Assurance Agency for Higher Education) 2007 Major review of healthcare programmes: final review trends report 2003-6. QAA.

Repper J, Breeze J 2007 User and carer involvement in the training and education of health professionals: a review of the literature. International Journal of Nursing Studies 44:511-519.

Simons L, Tee S, Lathlean J, Burgess A, Herbert L, Gibson C (2007) A socially inclusive approach to user participation in higher education. Journal of Advanced Nursing 58(3):246-255.

Smith E, Ross F, Donovan S 2008 Service user involvement in nursing, midwifery and health visiting research: a review of evidence and practice. International Journal of Nursing Studies 45(2):298-315.

Tew J, Gell C, Foster S 2004 Learning from experience: Involving service users and carers in mental health education and training. Higher Education Academy/NIMHE West Midlands/Trent Workforce Development Confederation, York.

Tyler G 2006 Addressing barriers to participation: service user involvement in social work training. Social Work Education 25(4):385-392.

Walmsley J, Johnson K 2003 Inclusive research with people with learning disabilities: past, present and futures. Jessica Kingsley Publishers, London.

Williams J 2005 Achieving meaningful inclusion for people with profound and multiple learning disabilities. Tizard Learning Disability Review 10(1):52.

Communication

Louise Talbott and Jane Parr

This chapter focuses on the importance of addressing communication issues when working towards inclusion for people with intellectual disabilities. An approach is put forward that helps us consider the different elements of inclusive communication. We examine some of the barriers to communication experienced by people with intellectual disabilities and how by addressing these barriers we can improve inclusion. It then shares some practical examples of how people with intellectual disabilities have been included in Leicester, Leicestershire and Rutland. The experience reported in the chapter is based upon working with a Specialist Learning Disability Service. Finally it will look at some ideas for the way forward and how we can work towards improving inclusion for people with the most complex communication needs.

OBJECTIVES

- To explain why communication is fundamental to achieving inclusion
- To consider what constitutes inclusive communication
- To explain the communication barriers experienced by people with intellectual disabilities in current methods of inclusion
- To demonstrate how users and carers can participate in the development of a communication strategy

KEY LEARNING POINTS

- The importance of good communication in achieving inclusion
- Why current approaches to inclusion may not be effective for many people with intellectual disabilities
- Approaches to improving communication and how these can be used to achieve inclusion

INCLUSION AND COMMUNICATION

Although many people with intellectual disabilities are now living in the community the evidence generated from people at consultation events locally and which will be reported within this chapter, suggests that they still do not on the whole feel listened to or included in decisions that are made about them. This makes them feel excluded and often lonely. Inclusion is more than just being located in the community it is about the contribution one makes being valued. It is about being able to make choices, grow in relationships, have the dignity of valued social roles and share with others, ordinary places and activities (O'Brien 1989).

Valuing People (2001) and its focus on the principles of rights, inclusion, independence and choice has significantly impacted on people's awareness of the lack of effective communication taking place with many people with intellectual disabilities.

Communication allows us to say what we would like from life, understand what is on offer to us, build relationships and contribute to the building of the local community and society as a whole.

Jones (2001) states that people with intellectual disabilities are frequently prevented from making even the first steps towards achieving these principles because they do not have the adequate means to do so. Nowhere is this truer than in the area of communication.

This chapter explores the idea of what 'adequate' means in order for people to achieve inclusion. It will explore the idea that inclusive communication is a social interaction where the giving and receiving of information achieves desired outcomes for those involved and facilitates social connection. The outcome may be getting something you want or letting someone know how you feel. Social connections are the relationships that people establish throughout their lifetimes that enable them to be regarded as a member of society. These may range from close relationships with friends and family or they may be passing connections such as a relationship with the local shopkeeper, bus driver or postman.

HOW TO ACHIEVE INCLUSIVE COMMUNICATION

In order to achieve inclusive communication consideration needs to be given to the context in which the communication takes place, the significance of having shared ways of giving and receiving information, and the importance of the style and quality of interaction.

If, when people communicate, they consider all three aspects of inclusive communication and make the necessary adjustments then people may achieve the social connections that allow them to be included.

1. The context

In order to achieve inclusive communication we need to ensure that the context supports the successful giving and receiving of information. The context consists of several elements.

The physical environment

Careful consideration is needed if the physical environment is to be supportive of communication; the exact requirements will depend on individual needs but would include ensuring that there are not too many distractions such as background noise, the lighting is good, the layout of the room and where people are positioned when they communicate supports effective communication and that there are visual clues that support understanding.

Timing

Communication can be affected by how much time you have available to either get your message across or listen to somebody else's message. Many people with intellectual disabilities require longer considering information and making their response.

It is particularly important for people who do not use formal systems of communication that there is understanding of how they express their views and time spent with them in a variety of situations to get a clear picture of their likes and dislikes. Even people who use formal systems may need information sending out before say a consultation event so that they can discuss it and therefore feel confident that they have understood the information and can give their views.

Another aspect of timing is how current the information is that is being talked about. With complex communication skills we can talk about things that have happened in the past and things that may happen in the future. Some people with intellectual disabilities cannot communicate about these abstract ideas and need to express their views by responding to things as they happen.

Opportunities

The environment needs to offer a range of opportunities to communicate, such as meeting new people, making choices and giving opinions. It is important that these opportunities are made accessible to people by considering the best ways of engaging each individual in them.

2. Shared ways of giving and receiving information

When we are thinking about people with intellectual disabilities it is necessary to recognise a wide range of behaviours as communication (Kelly 2000) and facilitate their use and understanding as part of everyday interactions; for example, people may walk away to show they want to finish a conversation or push a meal away to indicate they do not like it, alternatively they may tap their knee to indicate they need to use the toilet or lead someone to a place to communicate what they want. Some of these behaviours will be organised into what we may refer to as a language whereas some may be a unique combination of behaviours that one individual uses (Table 15.1).

Ensuring there are shared ways of communicating that support the giving and receiving of information is essential to inclusive communication. Choosing the best ways to do this will depend on the needs of the communicative partners involved. Whichever way is used there is also a need to consider how complicated the information is that is being presented. Factors that make information harder to understand include the length and structure

Table 15.1   Systems of communication

Type	Description	Examples
Formal systems	Organised and structured Used consistently by a group of people	Spoken languages Signing systems Symbol systems Objects of reference schemes
Individual systems	Unique to an individual Not necessarily recognised by others	Vocalisations Actions Behaviour
Supporting ways	Adds to the message Cultural May/may not be understood by others Can carry more weight than the primary system being used	Facial expression Interpersonal distance Body posture Gesture Tone of voice Volume

of sentences, the complexity of the words used and how easy the ideas are to understand. An example of this is the common mistake of trying to make written information easier to understand by adding pictures without considering the complexity of the language used or the message itself.

3. The style and quality of interaction

In order to achieve positive interactions an appropriate style needs to be adopted. The style of interaction reflects the values and beliefs held by the people communicating.

As part of inclusive communication there is a need to move towards a more supportive style of interaction where the expectation is that the individual can make choices, express opinions and make decisions even if this involves an element of risk. A caring style is appropriate in some situations but when enabling people to be included this more supportive style is required. Dowson & Bates (2004) speak of the difference between a supportive relationship and a caring one:

'Support is enabling whereas care is paternalistic, these contrasting attitudes translate of course into the aims and behaviours of the supporter within a relationship.'

We also need to ensure that we communicate in a way that shows we value the beliefs and culture of the other person and treat them with respect. This will vary depending on the nature of the relationship, for example communicative partners that know each other well may use more touch and stand closer.

In summary competent communicative partners with adequate means to facilitate inclusion can:

- Consider the context of the communication
- Choose and use the most appropriate style of interaction
- Use the best ways and level of communication to support and check out understanding
- Understand and respond to the ways people are using to express themselves

COMMUNICATION BARRIERS IN RELATION TO INCLUSION

1. The context

Physical environment

Ensuring the physical environment supports communication is very important. For example people with intellectual disabilities are more likely to have a sensory impairment than people who do not (Carvill 2001). Therefore barriers may include poor lighting, too much background noise and too many distractions. Equally, running consultation events in crowded halls or having an interview in a small room may immediately present a barrier for some people with intellectual disabilities.

A lack of resources in the environment can also cause barriers to inclusive communication, e.g. if an environment does not have a loop system (part of hearing assistive technology that enables people with hearing loss to hear better in group settings), access to picture materials or does not have suitable objects of reference then the ways in which people can communicate in that particular environment may be limited.

Timing

Many consultations that are carried out by services are one-off events either relating to a service that happened in the past or something planned for the future. This type of approach will present barriers to people who need to tell us about things as they happen. Including people with intellectual disabilities can take considerable time, as they may need longer to think about the information and have it repeated several times in order to form a view about it. Some people with intellectual disabilities may have to experience something in order to be able to communicate about it and more importantly they may only be able to tell you about something when they are actually experiencing the event. It has already been established that communication can be affected by how much time you have available to either get your message across or listen to somebody else's message; therefore if a support worker in a residential home or day service has a number of people to assist and a limited amount of time to do it in, it is unlikely they will have enough time to spend with someone if they try to strike up a conversation or express an opinion not relating to the task.

Opportunities

The need for the White Paper Valuing People suggests that in the past people with intellectual disabilities have not had adequate opportunities to express their views and be included in decisions about their lives. In the past many opportunities to include people were lost because information was not presented in a way that people understood. Other barriers have related to expectations linked to people's attitudes and values. If we do not value someone's opinion we are not going to seek it or act upon it. In the past people with intellectual disabilities were not expected to be able to make a valuable contribution and were physically excluded from society. There was little expectation that they could make choices about friends, partners, jobs and homes let alone how the NHS operates or who should run the country.

Jones reported that:

> 'under-occupation and subsequent low engagement in activity has often been observed in more institutional settings and that this did not always change in community settings. Higher engagement is associated with more positive contact from staff, which leads to more opportunities for communication.'

Jones 2000

2. Sharing ways

We know that approximately 80% of people with intellectual disabilities do not acquire effective speech and that many are unable to read and write (Foundation for People with Learning Disabilities figures, quoted in RCSLT 2006). If we focus only on speech and writing as ways of communicating we are potentially going to exclude the majority of people with intellectual disabilities.

In a western society the way information is shared tends to be through speaking and writing, often in a formal and complex way. For example, the way we usually find out what is going on in the community is through newspapers, leaflets, television and, increasingly, the Internet. The way we are encouraged to contribute is often through written surveys and formal consultation events. Similarly everyday interactions while shopping, going to the leisure centre or going to work are mainly conducted through spoken or written communication (Jones & Swift 1994).

Ruth Townsley (1998) argued that we live in a society that relies heavily upon the printed word to communicate with others and be informed about issues that affect us. She goes on to say:

> 'For the majority of people with learning disabilities however, a society that relies on printed information is a society that excludes them.'

Formal systems

Pease (1981) noted that research in the field of linguistics found that people higher up the social ladder tended to communicate using a greater variety and complexity of words and phrases. This has led society to associate power and status with people who are more articulate and give less value to other ways of communicating. Furthermore we complicate and confuse the message for those who share it by using abbreviations and jargon that inevitably exclude people. As a result there are still people today who find it hard to see that it takes more skill, and should therefore be more valued, to explain what you mean fully by using the most appropriate ways and level of complexity for the audience.

Individual systems

As individual systems are by definition unique to a particular person it is harder to interpret and respond to people who use these if you do not know them well. In practice much of the work of speech and language therapists in the past has focused on supporting others to identify and develop these individual systems. If society is going to include people who use individual systems there is a need to develop the use of communication passports or profiles that give information about the best ways of supporting the person to understand and express themselves. This will allow the individual to communicate with a greater range of people and for a picture of their preferences to be built up which allows them to contribute to decisions that are made that affect their lives.

There are many useful tools and techniques that can support people to communicate more effectively, such as talking mats, picture exchange systems and language development schemes. These systems have often been adopted in isolation as a universal solution without a clear understanding of an individual's or a group's specific needs. There needs to be greater understanding of these tools and which ones will be most useful in a given situation.

In the past carers and support workers have had limited access to training in communication skills and the best ways to support communication. Training tended to focus on specific methods such as signing rather than understanding how best to equip people with the adequate means to communicate inclusively. The introduction of the Learning Disability Award Framework (www.ldaf.org.uk) goes some way to addressing this as does much of the training in person centred approaches where communication is considered in all its forms in order to put the person at the centre of planning their lives.

The best approach to improving communication is not to expect to communicate the same way with everybody but to share a sophisticated level of awareness of communication and how to gauge other people's communicative needs so that one can then adapt to make each interaction as effective as possible.

3. The style and quality of interaction

Until fairly recently most people with intellectual disabilities were educated in separate schools, lived in isolated hospitals and homes and attended segregated day centres. This has been a barrier for a lot of people as they have experienced only a limited number of communication partners. This has limited the experiences of people with intellectual disabilities to build up a broader range of social connections but just as importantly it has not given the wider public a chance to build up positive relationships with people with intellectual disabilities.

The quality of any interaction relies on positive values and beliefs. Traditionally people with intellectual disabilities have been seen as people to care for and this has led to a style of communication that is controlling. Recent policy in relation to health and social care, for example 'Valuing People' (2001), 'Independence, Well Being and Choice' (2005) and 'Our Health, Our Care, Our Say' (2006), has seen an emphasis on shifting away from this view by focusing on involvement and choice.

The Mental Capacity Act (2005) has helped in establishing that people should be seen as having capacity to make life decisions unless proved otherwise. It supports the idea that we are entitled to make informed choices. This means that information needs to be presented in a way that enables individuals to weigh up the advantages and disadvantages of any decision.

Despite anti-discriminatory legislation the language that can be used in relation to people with intellectual disabilities is often still exclusionary.

Due to the barriers to inclusive communication it has often been difficult for people with intellectual disabilities to build up a wide range of social connections. Commonly their relationships have been limited to family and close friends; this is particularly true for people with individualised ways of communicating.

Seeing people with intellectual disabilities as people first leads to a willingness to spend time with them or listen to what they have to say. It is only by changing how we value people that we can develop more inclusive communication.

EXAMPLES OF WORKING TO REDUCE COMMUNICATION BARRIERS

Since the introduction of Valuing People (Department of Health 2001) and the current focus on involvement and choice in health and social care there is far more emphasis on gaining people's views and delivering more person centred services. Activities like meetings and consultation events have had to be more inclusive.

The initial approach to inclusive communication in Leicestershire, Leicester and Rutland in 2000 was the development of a Communication Strategy which would give the framework for all future work. This was based on an enabling model that aims to provide people with the knowledge, skills, resources, guidelines and support that they require to develop more inclusive communication. The strategy has been adopted by the three Learning Disability Partnership Boards in the areas identified and is continuing to be developed. The Partnership Boards were set up in response to Valuing People and consist of people with intellectual disabilities, family carers and statutory and voluntary services. Their role is to steer the learning disability agenda.

The implementation of the strategy includes making communication more inclusive in the following areas:

1. *To improve communication for an individual.* This includes ensuring that communication passports are developed for anyone that needs them. These will look at the best ways to help someone to understand and to express themselves. This work is particularly linked to the development of person centred plans and health action plans to ensure that people can be fully involved in these. Another priority is to work with people who are going through major life changes to ensure that they are as involved as possible in the decisions that are made.
2. *To improve communication in environments such as homes or places that people go to.* The focus will be on reducing the barriers to communication in these environments so that communication becomes more inclusive and people can be more involved in areas such as recruiting staff, choosing what to do and what not to do and making complaints.

3. *To improve communication with services.* Focusing on supporting services to produce information in ways that are easier to understand and improving involvement and consultation.

4. *To improve communication in communities.* Focusing on awareness raising and providing general advice.

The Communication Strategy is now called the 'Communication Plan'. More details can be found on the LDICN website.

The Speech and Language Therapy service in Leicestershire has been able to work with the Partnership Boards to ensure that inclusive communication has underpinned these initiatives. Examples of these projects are presented below. They show the attempts to ensure the breakdown of the communication barriers hindering inclusion for people with intellectual disabilities in these projects.

WORKING WITH THE PARTNERSHIP BOARDS

The Partnership Boards have developed a range of techniques to ensure people with intellectual disabilities are included as much as possible, these include:

- The use of advocates to support individual people to understand and contribute to the meetings
- Ensuring all papers are produced in a way that is easy to understand and are sent out early enough for people to have support to go through them and decide what they want to say about them
- The use of coloured cards so that people can say when they do not understand something and when they want to speak or ask questions
- Having less formal meetings and a chance to discuss things in smaller groups
- Writing up things that have been decided on flipchart, supported by pictures
- Reducing the number of items discussed and giving people more time to understand issues and make their comments
- Allowing times for self advocates to ask questions
- Having people with intellectual disabilities as co-chairs
- Having a briefing meeting before the main meeting

When interviewed, the co-chairs of one of the Partnership Boards (both people with intellectual disabilities) spoke of how the boards had impacted in their lives:

'The Partnership Boards are beginning to be all right...I think they need to do more communication training but it makes us involved...we are the co-chairs and we have learnt to speak up for everyone... about things like transport, day services and sometimes care and social services...we call people to come and speak to us... people listen and treat us better...it's made us confident ...we have more ideas of services...it helps to try and get what you want... meeting new people is good...I have a voice now.'

David & Donna

Communication

Although the Partnership Boards would all say there is more work to do the expectation is that people with intellectual disabilities have the most valuable contributions to make to the work of the boards and that if we remove the barriers to communication they can make these contributions more fully.

DEVELOPING GUIDELINES AND RESOURCES

In Leicester, Leicestershire and Rutland people with intellectual disabilities have been employed to help develop and check the resources and guidelines that have been developed.

Employing people with intellectual disabilities demonstrates the value their contribution to the planning and delivery of speech and language therapy services holds. It also develops positive social connections in a work situation. The insight they have given about the best ways to communicate with people is based on their first-hand experience of barriers to communication and this has influenced the emphasis of the work and the direction it has taken.

DELIVERING TRAINING

As part of the overall communication plan the 'learning plan' looks at opportunities to learn more about communication.

A similar approach to that of person-centred planning has been adopted. An introductory day covers the key aspects of communicating with people with intellectual disabilities and further learning opportunities look in more depth at the different aspects, such as signing and making written information easier to understand. There are two introductory days – one for staff who work with people with intellectual disabilities exclusively and a day for people who do not. The latter day explains more about how people with intellectual disabilities are excluded from the community and how inclusive communication can help to change this. This training has been delivered to local community services including firemen, council workers and vicars. Both days include learning about the context in which communication takes place, ways of communicating and positive styles of interaction as well as the barriers that may be encountered in each area.

People with intellectual disabilities are actively involved in the planning and delivery alongside other people who have volunteered to help. These volunteers include family carers and paid workers from the independent sector, health services and social care. Feedback has been positive and it is in its third year. Every year trainers and therapists spend a day together to check the material is up to date and to support one another.

Supporting hospital closure – working with advocates

The final long-stay hospital in Leicester was closed in 2006 and over 80 people were moved into the community, mainly in supportive living schemes. A large number were unfamiliar with the community and did not use formal ways of communicating. A team was set up to focus on the resettlement process including health and social care staff. There was input from the existing nursing staff; this was important as they had been the residents' main communicative

INTELLECTUAL DISABILITY AND SOCIAL INCLUSION

partners for years. Advocates were appointed to work alongside the nurses to gather and represent the residents' views in the decision making process. An advocate for carers was also appointed. Speech and Language Therapy were asked to support the process of involving the hospital residents.

A lot of thought went into where the best place to 'talk' to people about the move was. It varied for different individuals but for many it was in the choice of homes that was available to them.

People were supported to spend time in the community areas they were due to move into, interacting with local people and building up social connections.

People's experience of change varied and this was taken into account when planning how to involve each individual. For many it was important to communicate the things that were going to stay the same as much as the things that were going to change, e.g. family visits, personal belongings, outines, day care. Speech and Language Therapy worked closely with Psychology to think about how people might be able to express the many different emotions that change evokes.

Although the timing of the closure was known for a number of years for many people the best way of explaining what was about to happen and find out their views was through observing their reactions to events as they happened. It was inappropriate to give copious spoken, written or picture information about what was going to happen way in advance of the event. Some group events looking at pictures of properties and objects of reference such as suit cases and personal belongings were held but they were close to the actual event.

The success of the involvement is difficult to measure but from visiting people in their new homes it appears that for the majority of people the move was positive.

Consulting on day service modernisation

One of the earliest consultations that Speech and Language Therapy supported in Leicester was the consultation on modernising day services in Leicester. There were several barriers that needed to be overcome. The focus was on people with more formal ways of communicating although some information was gained by observing people to see what they enjoyed doing. Time was also spent talking to carers.

The formal consultation considered the context and what the modernisation of day services would mean for people who attended them. The main changes were considered to be the use of community facilities and more opportunities around employment. The first part of the planning was to look at what experiences people had in these areas so that they could say whether these were better or worse than the experiences they had in the day centres. A questionnaire was then developed based on these experiences using easy language supported by pictures and symbols. This was delivered by advocates and speech and language therapists who also used signing. There were checks to see if people were really understanding or were choosing the last item or saying everything was good. This avoided compliance, i.e. people wanting to please the questioners, and acquiescence, i.e. the tendency to say yes to everything.

Consulting on specialist intellectual disability and generic health services

The Local Management Team requested that the views of people with intellectual disabilities about health services were sought in order to inform the plans for integrating specialist intellectual disability health services with social services. Speech and Language Therapy, local advocacy services and a lead health facilitator ran two consultation days to find out what people with intellectual disabilities thought was good and bad about current services. This type of one-off event will only ever capture the views of people with formal systems of communication but activities were planned to try to make it as inclusive as possible. Supporters were identified who were skilled communicators and could enable individuals to understand or express their views. Most of the activities were carried out in small groups.

Techniques used included:

- Sending out information about the day in easy to understand formats
- Producing a timetable for the day that was supported by pictures and displayed throughout the day so that it could be continually referred to
- Rooms, facilitators, topics and people attending the day were allocated a colour. This enabled most people to independently know what was happening next and where they should be
- A range of approaches were used including discussions supported by pictures; acting out situations and asking people what they thought was good and bad; multi-media quizzes including familiar formats such as 'Who wants to be a millionaire'; presenting accessible health leaflets and multi-media information and asking for feedback on them; videoing individuals saying what they thought about health services they had experienced.

Criticisms of the day were based on transport to and from the venue, comments about refreshments and a lack of support from local day centres. A number of people asked why there were no doctors present. One person suggested a newsletter be produced and circulated to the day centres to keep people up to date and there were general comments about the need to keep on meeting to think about the future of health services.

Useful information from the day included that people still felt information was too complicated and that people with intellectual disabilities are not generally listened to in health services. There was agreement that although they wanted information to be in easy words and pictures they did not want lots of graphic pictures of medical procedures as this would be too much. They said that they would like to have more say about how they are cared for and be more involved in the decisions about their health. They said they would like to be treated as adults. People showed they understood a lot about how to eat healthily but that they wanted the right to choose what they eat. The group said there were not enough activities they could get to, to keep fit.

Following these events the information was presented to the Partnership Boards and the NHS Trust. The Trust now has an advisory group who meet regularly to discuss the development of health services. People with intellectual disabilities and their carers take an active part in this group.

CONCLUSION – THE WAY FORWARD

Although there is room to improve the way people who can use formal ways of communicating are involved, consideration urgently needs to be given to how we involve people who use individual systems. They need opportunities in their everyday lives to express what they think about a variety of issues. The evidence about what they like and dislike needs to be recorded in person-centred plans and communication passports so that everyone can act upon it and use the evidence to help plan and evaluate services.

There is a need to ensure that people are really included and not just consulted with – people have often reported that they are fed up with being asked what they want because afterwards they cannot see any changes.

There needs to be an increased awareness of how to make inclusive communication work and an effort to develop communicative competence that will support people with intellectual disabilities to develop their skills and confidence to build up a wider range of social connections and become valued members of the community. For this to happen there needs to be learning opportunities and good quality resources that support people's communication. These need to be shared across the country so time is not wasted duplicating work and the real act of including people can happen.

ACKNOWLEDGEMENTS

The examples given in this chapter have taken place in Leicester, Leicestershire and Rutland and have been led by the Leicestershire Partnership Trust Speech and Language Therapy Service and other members of the City and Counties Communication Groups and Partnership Boards.

REFERENCES

Carvill S 2001 Review: sensory impairments, intellectual disability and psychiatry. Journal of Intellectual Disability Research 45:467-483.

Department of Health 2001 Valuing People: a new strategy for learning disability for the 21st century. The Stationery Office, London.

Department of Health 2005 Independence, Well Being and Choice: Our Vision for the Future of Social Care for Adults in England. Cm 6499. The Stationery Office, London.

Department of Health 2006 Our Health, Our Care, Our Say: a new direction for community services. Cm 6737. The Stationery Office, London.

Dowson S, Bates P 2004 Triangles of support: creating relationships that support inclusion. An emerging themes paper. www.ndt.org.uk (accessed 30.05.07).

Jones J 2000 A total communication approach towards meeting the communication needs of people with learning disabilities. Tizard Learning Disability Review 5(1).

Jones J 2001 The communication gap: a paper exploring the fundamental nature of communication in achieving the 'New Vision' of the White Paper 'Valuing People.' www.learningdisabilities.org.uk (accessed 3/2/07).

Jones J, Swift P 1994 Communication as a priority in services for people with learning disabilities. Social Services Research 1994 – 1, The University of Birmingham.

Kelly A 2000 Working with adults with learning disabilities. Winslow Press Ltd, Bicester.

Learning Disability Awards Framework 2003. Commission for Social Care Inspection, London. www.ldaf.org.uk (accessed 7/3/08).

Mental Capacity Act (2005) www.mentalcapacityact.com (accessed 7/3/08).

O'Brien John 1989 What's worth working for: Leadership for better quality human services. Responsive Systems Associates thechp@syr.edu.

Parr J 2006 Making communication better: the communication plan for adults with learning disabilities in Leicester, Leicestershire and Rutland. www.ldicn.org.uk (accessed 7/3/08).

Pease A 1981 Body language: how to read others' thought through their gestures. Sheldon Press, London.

RCSLT 2006 Communicating quality 3.

Townsley R 1998 Information is power. In: Ward L (ed) The impact of accessible information on people with learning disabilities. Innovations in advocacy and empowerment for people with intellectual disabilities. Lisieux Hall Publications, Chorley.

INDEX

Index

Index